David Jenkins

Listening to Gynaecological Patients' Problems

Springer-Verlag
London Berlin Heidelberg New York
Paris Tokyo

David Jenkins, MD, FRCOG
Erinville Hospital, Western Road, Cork, Eire

Front Cover: Ivory female diagnostic statuette, reproduced by permission of The
Wellcome Institute Library, London

ISBN 3-540-16207-0 Springer-Verlag Berlin Heidelberg New York
ISBN 0-387-16207-0 Springer-Verlag New York Berlin Heidelberg

Library of Congress Cataloging-in-Publication Data
Jenkins, David, 1936-
Listening to gynaecological patients.
Includes bibliographies and index. 1. Genito-urinary organs – Diseases – Diagnosis.
2. Generative organs, Female – Diseases – Diagnosis. 3. Gynecologist and patient.
4. Interpersonal communication. I. Title. [DNLM: 1. Communication. 2. Genital
Diseases, Female – diagnosis. 3. Physician-Patient Relations. WP 141 J52L]
RG107.J46   1986   618.1'075   86-20200
ISBN 0-387-16207-0 (U.S.)

Filmset by Tradeset Photosetting, Welwyn Garden City, Hertfordshire.
Printed by Page Bros (Norwich) Limited, Mile Cross Lane, Norwich

2128/3916-543210

£ 6·80

This book is to be returned on or before the last date stamped below.

-7. JAN. 1991

8 DEC 1988

6 FEB 1991

10 DEC 1991

APR 1992

JAN. 1993

APR 1993

11 JAN. 1994

FEB. 1994

1994

1994

-8 JAN 1996

22 FEB 1996

14 MAY 1997

22 DEC 2000

20·6·03

Preface

Gynaecological textbooks generally are divided into sections according to pathological diagnoses, not according to symptoms or symptom complexes. Students of gynaecology, because they initially acquire information from textbooks, are conditioned by the organisation of these texts to think of gynaecology in terms of pathological entities rather than symptom complexes. Gynaecological patients, however, do not present complaining of endometriosis or endometrial malignancy or hypophyseal–ovarian dysfunction; rather they present with symptoms like 'pain low down in the tummy', 'bleeding from the front passage' or 'irregular periods'.

This book attempts to help students of gynaecology (including everyone from students learning the subject for the first time, through family doctors, to hospital doctors of all grades) to approach their patients as people, as distinct from possible pathological entities, to listen to them, and to communicate with them. In order to help achieve this, the text is divided according to symptoms or related groups of symptoms. Within each division, pertinent questions are listed in the words that might be used in addressing a patient, followed by a key explaining the significance of the questions and a brief discussion of the problems of the condition under consideration. It is hoped that this approach will facilitate the taking and interpretation of case histories, thus aiding differential diagnosis and clinical management, and will initiate the process of self-teaching.

The book tries to emphasise that, especially in gynaecology, the same symptom (e.g. heavy periods) may have very different significance in different patients in terms of diagnosis and management.

I am content that the exercise has not been marred by the blind conviction of a crusader but is often characterised by the hesitancy of someone who knows he could well be wrong and is anxious to learn by his mistakes.

Acknowledgements

I want to thank whoever taught me to say 'I don't understand' when I didn't, and those of my teachers who taught me how to think rather than rely upon dogma and 'fact'. Hiding ignorance behind labels is common in medicine. The medical student is bombarded with dogma, 'facts' and labels and rarely has time to ask questions. He is too often programmed rather than educated, an unfortunate fate for some of our brightest school leavers. I thank those students who refused to accept, without question, my dogma and made me think as I shared knowledge with them.

I wish to thank my secretaries, Miss Bridget Barrett and Miss Maureen Gleeson, who over the past 7 years have produced draft after draft of this simple text, helping to bring some order out of confusion.

Finally, particular thanks are due to Michael Jackson of Springer, who has performed in a manner highly reminiscent of an obstetrician in his antepartum and intrapartum care of this parturient.

Cork, Eire   David Jenkins
June 1986

Contents

Communication Between Patient and Doctor 1

How to Proceed 7

Stage I: What Type of Problem Is It?
    Classification by Symptoms 9

Stage II: Background History 11

Stage III: Consideration in More Detail
    of the Presenting Problem 13

Category A Menstrual Problems and Abnormal Bleeding 15

Category B Urinary Problems 43

Category C Uterovaginal Prolapse 49

Category D Abdominal Pain 53

Category E Abdominal Distension or Mass 57

Category F Vaginal Problems 61

Category G Difficulty with Intercourse 71

Category H Fertility Problems 75

Category I Family Planning Problems 83

Category J Psychosexual Problems 87

Category K Hirsutism 93

Category L Menopausal Problems 97

Epilogue 100

Index 101

Communication Between Patient and Doctor

Although the student cannot understand disease without understanding pathology, when it comes to clinical practice the input
from the patient is a symptom. It follows that although the doctor
should know which pathologies may cause a particular symptom,
it is more efficient for him to think from the symptom to the list of
pathologies which cause that symptom. Again, it is more efficient
because it 'programs' the doctor's 'computer' to respond to
symptoms, which is the information he deals in with his patient. If
we take the example of pelvic pain, it is simpler to learn a list of
causes of pelvic pain than to review a list of pathologies, searching
through the symptoms associated with them to see whether or not
these include pelvic pain.

This approach to gynaecology, commencing from symptoms,
helps effective and efficient communication with patients and
problem solving. The cost, in medical, emotional and financial
terms, of communication failure between doctor and patient is very
high. It is understandable that the patient, who may be anxious,
sometimes fails to listen to the doctor. It is unacceptable that the
doctor does not listen to the patient (Fig. 1).

Taking some examples, the severity and nature of pain present
many problems in terms of communication; how accurately can the
doctor assess the patient's complaint of heavy periods or the severity of her dysmenorrhoea? Again, a patient may present with a

The Patient

Fear

Forgetfulness

Frustration

Illness

etc.

The Doctor

Haste

Ignorance

Indifference

Fatigue

Prejudice

etc.

Fig. 1. Factors which might interfere with history taking and giving.

complaint of vaginal discharge, which may be secondary, her real problem being psychosexual. Unless the doctor is listening for clues that suggest the latter, he may pointlessly and expensively pursue the treatment of a non-existent vaginal discharge whilst losing the respect of his patient, who finds it too embarrassing to discuss the underlying major sexual problem.

Remember that the patient may be trying to tell you more than is contained in the words she is using. She may also be asking you questions which she does not verbalise. This makes it even more important to get the verbal communication as clear and precise as possible.

The doctor must consequently know which questions to ask (i.e. those relevant to a presenting complaint), know what the questions mean to himself and to the patient, and appreciate the significance of the answers. The student's own appreciation of the questions is, of course, based on his understanding of the relevant physiology, anatomy, pathology, biochemistry etc., without which the questions would be meaningless.

The questions suggested as appropriate in this book are not meant as a crutch for non-thinking doctors, replacing a proper understanding of the underlying pathology, but as an aide-mémoire so that interviews can proceed in a relaxed but precise way and the doctor has time to register the important non-verbal information available to him and to develop rapport. If one goes for a walk by the sea one is unlikely to enjoy the view if one has to concentrate on how to put one foot in front of the other. The view is the totality of the patient's problems. The questions are the steps you take in coming to understand those problems. Rapport is sharing the view with the patient. Is she frightened, indifferent, depressed, lonely, shallow, shy, hating or enjoying having to be in the position she is in? How would you feel in her situation? Rapport depends upon a sense of sharing. Doctors can bully patients into agreeing that they have almost any symptom in the book; which woman can deny that she has ever had a single episode of stress incontinence? Some patients need to be kept to the point during the interview, others need considerable time to expand their answers. If they are not given time, only half or even a false picture will emerge.

It is in my view one of the functions of medical teachers to make 'their students' at least adequate communicators. Expensive equipment is not necessary. Asking individual students to take their histories from patients in front of their colleagues quickly highlights talents and defects in communication technique. Getting the patient then to ask the student for an explanation of her problem and how it is to be managed is also highly revealing of communication skills.

In the context of this book, the 'lay' words used in the questionnaires are deliberately chosen so that most patients will understand the questions; 'tummy' is used for abdomen if the latter seems likely to prove difficult for the patient to understand. These questionnaires are also meant to help communication by clearly defining what factual information is necessary for differential diagnosis. The doctor cannot really listen to the patient if he is trying to remember what are the relevant questions he should be asking. Time must be allowed for assessment of how the patient responds to the questions, as this is an important help in evaluation. It is necessary to appreciate that some patients exaggerate and others minimise the severity of their symptoms and what causes them to do so. The importance of the history and the intelligent and informed interpretation of the history cannot be overemphasised and this is what this book is about (Fig. 2). Clinical examination and other investigations are not given emphasis here. Investigations such as laparoscopy and ultrasound have made considerable contributions to problem solving in gynaecology. They have not, and should not, replace a good history.

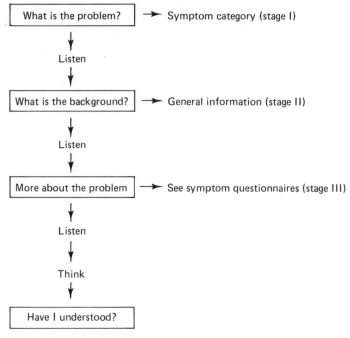

Fig. 2. Plan for history taking.

A Note on Exposition: The Second Half of Communication

Some patients like to feel they are making the decisions because they feel threatened and vulnerable if they 'hand over the reins' totally to the doctor. It is helpful in this situation if the doctor adopts the passive role and says things like "in all the circumstances do you feel that you should have your uterus or womb removed"? Any tendency to the "just take it from me, get shot of it" approach with this sort of patient is likely to stir up aggressive vibrations and should be avoided. Again, other patients prefer not to be responsible for decisions for many various reasons and they need to be told gently and firmly that the best course of action is this or that and they needn't worry and you will go ahead and organise everything. There are as many different approaches as there are patients, and most doctors either adopt a fairly innocuous 'middle of the road' blanket approach that offends or obtrudes minimally or naturally and appropriately change approach without thinking. It may be argued that as long as the surgeon or physician does a good job, an ill-natured grunt is as good as anything. Those who argue that way have never been patients, certainly not lay patients without any knowledge of the mysteries and horrors of medicine. The same factors that interfere with history taking can reduce the quality of exposition.

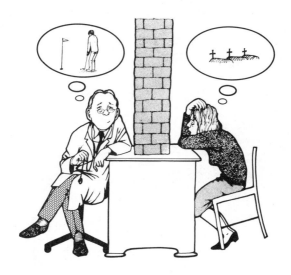

"Ye that have ears to hear . . ."

How to Proceed

Stage I

First, one should list the patient's symptoms in order of importance and under the main and subsidiary categories A-L (see index on pp. 9–10).

Stage II

The general background information is then obtained.

Stage III

Specific questions relating to the patient's particular problems are asked, as shown in each subcategory, e.g. A1, A2 etc.

This approach achieves three things with regard to the presenting complaint:

1. It *focuses* it
2. It *qualifies* it
3. It *evaluates* it

Stage I: What Type of Problem Is It? Classification by Symptoms

The following classification according to symptom complexes determines the questions to be asked; these are found at the start of each section later in the book (pp. 15–99).

CATEGORY A Menstrual Problems and Abnormal Bleeding

1. Failure of Periods to Start
2. Cessation of Periods
3. Abnormal (Heavy or Irregular) Periods
4. Painful Periods
5. Vaginal Bleeding After the Menopause
6. Vaginal Bleeding Before Puberty
7. Vaginal Bleeding During Pregnancy

CATEGORY B Urinary Problems

1. Urinary Incontinence
2. Other Bladder Problems

CATEGORY C Uterovaginal Prolapse

CATEGORY D Abdominal Pain

CATEGORY E Abdominal Distension or Mass

CATEGORY F Vaginal Problems

1. Pain in or Around the Vagina
2. Vulval Swelling
3. Discharge from the Vagina
4. Itching Around the Vulva
5. Warts Around the Vulva

CATEGORY G Difficulty with Intercourse

CATEGORY H Fertility Problems

1. Difficulty in Becoming Pregnant for the First Time
2. Difficulty in Becoming Pregnant Despite Previous Pregnancy
3. Difficulty in Having a Baby Because of Repeated Miscarriages

CATEGORY I Family Planning Problems

CATEGORY J Psychosexual Problems

CATEGORY K Hirsutism

CATEGORY L Menopausal Problems

Stage II: *Background History*

After noting the main and subsidiary problems the following basic information is required:

Is your general health good?

Is your weight steady/falling/rising?

Have you ever been pregnant?

If 'yes', how many pregnancies have you had in all?

How many living children do you have now?

When was your last child born?

      Day   Month   Year

Have you ever been referred to a gynaecologist before?

When was it?

What was it for and what treatment did you receive?

Are you having sexual intercourse?

If 'yes':

a) Since when have you been having sexual intercourse?

b) Would you be quite happy to find yourself pregnant?

c) If you are not on the pill do you or your husband use any form of contraception?

d) If 'yes' which form of contraception do you use — coil (IUD)/ cap/sheath/other?

If you smoke cigarettes, how many per day?

Are there any other factors at all you wish to mention?

This is an 'easy' section of the interview when the patient can be put at ease: you can look at her as distinct from writing down details of answers as you go along, notice how she is dressed, how she sits, her hands, her mood, her accent and whether she looks you in the eye. Open yourself to impressions and don't come too quickly to conclusions as to the sort of woman she is.

Stage III: Consideration in More Detail of the Presenting Problem

Questions relating to the category or subcategory of problem identified during stage I are posed. Answers are interpreted in the light of the key to these questions and the more general discussion contained within the sections entitled 'The Problem'.

Some questions will be redundant in certain circumstances. Relevant negative answers may be diagnostically important.

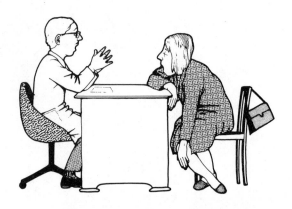

"The Niagara Falls wouldn't be in it, Doctor."

Category A Menstrual Problems and Abnormal Bleeding

A1
Failure of Periods to Start

*

Questions

1. Was anyone else in your family late starting their periods?
2. Are you smaller than your friends of the same age?
3. Did your breasts develop at the same age as the other girls in your school class?
4. Have you had difficulty starting to pass water recently?
5. Do you have monthly attacks of tummy pain?
6. Have you ever had a period brought on by tablets?

Key to Questions

Question 1. Delayed menarche is to some extent familial. If there is a familial factor, it would be preferable to be conservative and observe the situation.

Question 2. Primary amenorrhoea may be associated with small stature. This rapidly distinguishes two major groups: those with and those without a chromosomal factor.

Question 3. Is puberty normal? For example, is there any evidence of oestrogen deficiency (delayed or absent breast development; absence of pubic and axillary hair)?

Questions 4, 5. Cryptomenorrhoea due to imperforate hymen may cause these symptoms.

Question 6. Is there a normal uterus, a responsive endometrium and a normal anatomical passage from the uterine cavity to the vulva? If so, progesterones will induce a withdrawal bleed.

The Problem

The problem is that of primary amenorrhoea. The first question is — is it really a problem? The answer is that after the age of 16 it is probably worth investigating the situation if the patient is concerned enough to come to you for advice about it. Does the patient have normally developed sexual characteristics or not? If she has, exclude imperforate hymen by gentle examination and confirm normal vagina and uterus. This may require examination under anaesthesia. If secondary sexual characteristics are absent then a buccal smear and chromosome studies need to be carried out after reassuring the patient and arranging for determinations of plasma FSH and oestrogens. If the results of the chromosome studies are normal and FSH levels are high then either gonadal dysgenesis, resistant ovary syndrome or auto-immune oophoritis is likely to be present. If FSH levels are low, primary pituitary failure may be present. Hypothyroidism, pulmonary stenosis and coeliac disease are conditions to consider. Heterosexual characteristics may denote adrenal or ovarian tumour, congenital adrenal hyperplasia or abnormal presence of a Y chromosome (see Fig. 3).

Management

Psychological treatment involves a one to one relationship with the patient. These patients need a confidential personal relationship. One should see them oneself each time they come to the surgery or out-patient department. The absence of periods is less worrying for

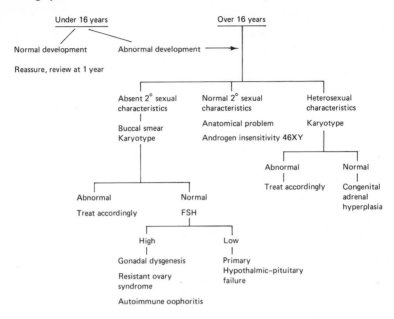

Fig. 3. Primary amenorrhoea. Plan of investigation.

patients than the short stature and poor breast development. These patients want to look normal. Oestrogens will achieve growth and breast development. Premature closure of epiphyses is not a problem and endometrial malignancy, which potentially is a problem, can be prevented by adding a progestogen to the oestrogen in the second half of the cycle.

Leave long-term anxieties aside and gain rapport by reassuring the patient that she will grow and breast development can be achieved. The fact that the patient will never be able to become pregnant can wait for another day and reassurance that her sex life will be normal is supportive.

Patients with Y chromosome in their karyotype are at increased risk of gonadal malignancy. The degree of risk may be as high as 30%. This indicates surgical removal of these gonads and the sooner this is done, the better. The psychological damage caused by clitoral enlargement in a girl of 12 or 13 with a mosaicism and Y chromosome might have been prevented if her gonads had been removed earlier. Remember that in testicular feminisation syndrome or androgen insensitivity syndrome the patient is a 46XY gonadal male with female phenotype, blind-ending vagina and no uterus. Testes may be palpable in the groins or upper labia or be intra-abdominal. Again, orchidectomy is indicated because of the cancer risk, which increases with age but is variably quoted as between 5% and 30%. Orchidectomy should, however, be deferred until full secondary sexual development has occurred. Oestrogen replacement with ethinyloestradiol 0.02 mg daily has been recommended. No anxiety about endometrial malignancy exists. Marked loss of libido following orchidectomy may occur. Vaginoplasty for the short vagina is rarely, if ever, necessary.

Further Reading

Dewhurst J (1984) Female puberty and its abnormalities. Churchill Livingstone, Edinburgh
Hawkins DF (ed) (1981) Gynaecological therapeutics, Chap. 1. Genetic and congenital sexual disorders. Bailliere Tindall, London

A2
Cessation of Periods

*

Questions

1. How long is it since your last period?
2. Have you notice any breast tingling or discomfort?
3. Have you noticed any sickness or nausea?
4. Have you noticed any abdominal swelling?
5. Did you have intercourse about the time of your last period?
6. a) Have you been on the pill?
   b) If 'yes', how long ago did you stop taking it?
7. Have you noticed any abnormal secretion from the breast?
8. Have you had any bad headaches recently?
9. Have you had disturbance of your vision?

10. Have you had spells without periods in the absence of pregnancy before?
11. Have you noticed any increased hair growth recently?
12. Have you noticed any falling-out of your scalp hair recently?
13. Have you noticed any change in your voice?
14. Were you on a weight-reducing diet when the periods stopped?
15. Were you unhappy for any reason when your periods stopped?
16. Have you had a recent pregnancy associated with haemorrhage?
17. Have you had a scrape or curettage recently?

Key to Questions

Question 1. Secondary amenorrhoea of more than 9 months' duration is not due to pregnancy.

Questions 2–5. Relate to the possibility of pregnancy.

Question 6. Relates to post-pill amenorrhoea as the cause of the problem.

Questions 7–9. Relate to hyperprolactinaemia.

Question 10. Refers to previous 'axis' dysfunction.

Questions 11–13. A positive answer suggests excess androgen production.

Question 12. Considers the possibility of thyroid disease being a factor.

Question 14. Considers weight-related factors influencing periods.

Question 15. Serves to assess whether emotional and psychological factors are involved.

Question 16. Refers to Sheehan's syndrome.

Question 17. Considers Asherman's syndrome.

The Problem

The first important diagnosis to exclude is pregnancy; the second most common cause is cortico-hypothalamic dysfunction, and the third, some dysfunction of the hypothalamic-hypophyseal-ovarian axis. Post-pill amenorrhoea, hyperprolactinaemia and premature menopause are other possibilities to bear in mind in secondary amenorrhoea. Careful enquiry about eating habits and weight change may reveal borderline or frank anorexia.

On general examination attention must be given to the following questions: What is the patient's affect? Is she under stress, and if so, what stress? Is there evidence of recent weight loss or gain? Does she look ill? Is there any evidence of endocrinopathy, thyroid disease, or hirsutism? Is there evidence of breast changes or galactorrhoea? Is there any abdominal mass (pregnancy, ovarian tumour)?

Bimanual examination excludes pregnancy, ovarian tumour and other pelvic diseases. A pituitary mass is excluded by radiology of the pituitary fossa and arrangements should be made for plasma prolactin, oestrogens and plasma FSH, LH and thyroxine to be measured.

Management

If the diagnosis is not one of pregnancy then reassure the patient about the common nature of secondary amenorrhoea. A search for precipitating psychological factors, and then an explanation that once you have excluded some unlikely but important possibilities you will await spontaneous recovery, unless pregnancy is desired, is usually what is required. Remember that to be told a skull X-ray is necessary is a fairly frightening thing.

Secondary amenorrhoea due to emotional upset requires only reassurance together with patient and commonsense support and advice in most cases. Imminent or frank psychosis obviously calls for specialised care; frank psychosis is not infrequently missed by referring doctors who have focussed on the presenting symptom and have immediately sought an organic/endocrinal cause. Stress-induced hyperprolactinaemia is a likely cause, and young teenagers doing exams under severe pressure sometimes present with secondary amenorrhoea. Letting them talk it out helps as long as you listen to patients and 'share their vulnerability'.

Anorectics require psychiatric help in some cases but others who are merely 'flirting' with the idea can be counselled and told that once they regain weight their periods will return. Hyperprolactinaemia may be treated by bromocriptine or surgical excision of prolactinomas in some cases. Oestrogen- or androgen-secreting tumours will require surgical treatment. Sheehan's syndrome requires gonadatrophin therapy if pregnancy is desired, whilst fitting a Dalcon Shield IUD after breaking down adhesions has been recommended for dealing with amenorrhoea due to Asherman's syndrome.

In summary (Fig. 4): Don't forget the possibility of pregnancy; remember that transient emotional stress causing amenorrhoea is very common; think about hyperprolactinaemia and weight change; and make sure that the patient does not have a hormone-secreting ovarian malignancy. Most patients with post-pill amenorrhoea recover spontaneously within 1 year and therapy for infertility subsequently is much more successful than was originally thought.

THINK FROM TOP DOWNWARDS

Pregnancy

Stress

Weight change

Post-pill

Axis dysfunction

Malignancy (must be excluded)

Hyperprolactinaemia

Other endocrinopathy

Drugs

Post-haemorrhage

Post-scrape

Fig. 4. Possible causes of secondary amenorrhoea.

Further Reading

Spenoff L, Glass RH, Kase NG (1978) Clinical gynaecological endocrinology and infertility, 2nd edn. Williams and Wilkins, Baltimore, p 97 ff

A3
Abnormal (Heavy or Irregular) Periods

*

Questions

1. For how long have you had this trouble?
2. Do you have regular monthly periods?
   If 'no':
   a) Are your periods occurring more often than once a month?
   b) Is there more than a month between your periods?
   c) What is the shortest time from the start of one period to the start of the next?
   d) What is the longest time from the start of one period to the start of the next?
3. Do you think your periods are too heavy?
   If 'yes':
   a) How many packets of pads/tampons do you require to use per period?
   b) Do you use double pads?
   c) Do you have 'floodings' which you cannot control?
   d) Are your everyday activities interfered with?
   e) Have you been taking iron in any form?
4. Do your periods last longer than normal?
   If 'yes': For how many days do they last?
5. Do you have bleeding between your periods?
   If 'yes':
   a) Does it usually occur midway between your periods?
   b) Does it occur after intercourse?
6. Have you had similar troubles in the past?
   If 'yes': Have you previously had a curettage (D&C or scraping of the womb)?
7. Have you had drugs, 'the pill' or other hormones for this trouble?
   If 'yes': Were they effective?
8. Would you like further children?

Key to Questions

Most of these questions are directed at precise definition of the menstrual dysfunction, duration and severity. The importance of this cannot be over-emphasised.

Question 6. Seeks information about previous similar problems, and previous diagnosis.

Question 7. Previous treatment with hormones is important. Patients are often ignorant of what treatment they have been given and why; often it has been inappropriate.

Question 8. Treatment possibilities depend upon whether the patient wants to retain her reproductive function.

The importance of these questions lies in the fact that a decision regarding hysterectomy may be made solely upon the patient's subjective assessment of her menstrual loss (and usually is). Most women who proceed to hysterectomy have no organic disease and haemoglobin levels in the normal range. It follows that the doctor's advice as to whether or not hysterectomy is indicated depends heavily on his evaluation of symptoms.

The Problem

Patients need guidance in defining precisely what their menstrual disturbance is. Menstrual bleeding needs to be clearly distinguished from non-menstrual bleeding. Postcoital bleeding may need to be offered as a possible symptom because the patient would decline to report this voluntarily. Menstrual problems can cause considerable misery, discomfort and inconvenience. They are amenable to effective treatment.

With regard to patients whose complaint is that their periods are heavier than normal, try to establish to what extent this is true. The average amount of blood lost at menstruation by different women has been estimated to be of the order of 40 ml, and losses heavier than 80 ml are considered abnormally heavy. However, there are considerable variations in what women themselves consider to be abnormally heavy. For example, women who have had tubal ligation might find the inconvenience of any menstrual loss to be such that they consider their loss to be too great, when, in fact, it is no heavier than normal. Menstrual loss is commonly heavier in

women with IUDs and they should be advised of this before the
IUD is decided upon as a method of contraception. Patients complaining of heavy menstrual bleeding with the device may be considering requesting sterilisation and this should be borne in mind
as well in the management of the problem.

The only absolute objective guide to the extent of the menstrual
loss is actually to collect all the towels or tampons used by the
patient and to measure the blood loss. This has been done in certain
experimental situations and considerable variation is seen in the
amount of blood lost between women who say that they have a
heavy loss; that is, some women complaining of a very heavy loss
are in fact found to have a small total loss compared with other
women who state that they have a normal loss. It is important,
therefore, to realise that there are two separate problems; firstly the
woman who indeed has a very heavy loss, associated with anaemia
and a direct threat to her health, and secondly the woman who
claims she has a heavy loss but in fact does not have such a heavy
loss as to influence her general health adversely. In the second
group, the woman is saying that she has a menstrual loss which
she considers too heavy and too inconvenient for her, and this also
needs to be treated. In extreme cases a measure of the haemoglobin
concentration will distinguish clearly between these two groups;
patients with haemoglobin below 70% can indeed be considered
as having menstrual loss greater than is consistent with continued
good health and direct treatment should be administered to prevent continuation of this loss. This situation can be masked by the
patient taking oral iron therapy to compensate for the blood loss
and this must be taken into consideration as well.

It is again necessary to get a precise history from patients who
complain that their periods are prolonged, because occasionally
these patients are complaining of bleeding during the last week of
a cycle which is then followed by the start of the 'proper' period. In
this situation there is an early shedding of some part of the
endometrium due to progestogen deficiency, so-called deficient
luteal phase bleeding. This is usually characterised by the onset of
intermittent brown staining some 3 weeks after the first day of the
last period, followed by the onset of what the patient often recog-
nises as the first day of the 'proper' period some 6 or 7 days after the
brown staining commences. In other patients the bleeding is virtu-
ally continuous throughout the cycle; in this situation it is very
likely that there is either some organic cause or failure of adequate
oestrogenic stimulation of the endometrium followed by an
inadequate progesterone stimulus, and these should be looked for.

A common problem is breakthrough bleeding on the contraceptive pill; this is usually easily remedied by increasing the progestogenic potency of the combined preparation. Some women have slight blood staining at the time of ovulation, 14 days before the first day of the next period. Ask particularly of the group of patients with intermenstrual bleeding whether the bleeding occurs after intercourse, because if this is the case one has to exclude carcinoma of the cervix before considering any other possibility.

In summary, with regard to menstrual irregularity or menstrual problems it is important to get a precise history as to what the menstrual irregularity or problem is; this may require time and patience on the part of the doctor. One should then distinguish between patients who have a 'real' menstrual problem, likely to have a hormonal or organic base, and patients whose periods are not abnormal but are saying that their periods are inconvenient and troublesome and that they want something done about either regulating, reducing or completely stopping them. Often when a woman who presents with menstrual problems has completed her family and finds various forms of contraception inconvenient, it may be that she is asking for either sterilisation and/or hysterectomy, and it is important to keep in mind that as many as 20% of patients who have tubal ligation carried out as a form of sterilisation return to gynaecologists soon thereafter, requesting hysterectomy.

In women at or about the menopause endometrial carcinoma has to be seriously considered before any other possible explanation of their menstrual disturbance is sought. However, in the younger woman the diagnosis is very much more likely to be some hormonal imbalance; in these patients, endometrial biopsy is not mandatory and the use of hormonal therapy to control menstrual irregularity is much more sensible than performing routine curettage and hoping that this will have therapeutic value.

Understanding and Correcting Uterine Haemorrhage

Students have always found it difficult to understand dysfunctional uterine haemorrhage and it has remained a vague entity in the minds of teachers as well as students. It is helpful to try to get a clear idea of hypothalamic–pituitary–ovarian interaction, for by understanding the mechanisms of dysfunction at these three levels it is possible to understand various menstrual irregularities (see Fig. 5).

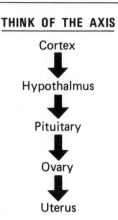

THINK OF THE AXIS

Cortex

Hypothalmus

Pituitary

Ovary

Uterus

1. Each unit of the axis can malfunction.

2. Feedback mechanisms between units of the axis can malfunction.

3. Multiple inputs into the axis can cause malfunction of the axis. These may be congenital, metabolic, endocrine, inflammatory, traumatic, neoplastic etc.

4. Dysfunctional uterine haemorrhage refers to malfunction <u>not</u> associated with organic disease.

Fig. 5. Understanding menstrual problems.

Seen in simple terms there are two feedback mechanisms between the ovary and the pituitary, one negative, one positive: Firstly, rising oestrogen levels in the follicular phase act by negative feedback to inhibit FSH release from the pituitary. Secondly, there is a pre-ovulatory oestrogen peak which brings about a release of LH from the pituitary, the so-called LH surge, and this is the positive feedback mechanism. Both negative and positive mechanisms may fail completely or be deficient and malfunction. This can result in, for example, prolonged anovulatory cycles with heavy bleeding because there has been no progesterone influence on the endometrium secondary to a failed positive feedback mechanism. In failed negative feedback mechanisms the FSH is not switched off and its continued stimulation of the ovary, although probably at a declining intensity, results in irregular cycles with abnormal bleeding. Another example of feedback mechanism dysfunction is the so-called deficient luteal phase in which the endometrium starts to shed prior to the start of the proper period; this probably occurs because of progesterone deficiency due to inadequate follicular development during the proliferative phase.

In terms of investigation of dysfunctional uterine bleeding, one first wants to know whether the ovary is producing oestrogen in reasonable quantities. This can be assessed either by measuring the plasma oestrogen levels or by giving the patient a progestogen for 5 days and then stopping this and seeing if any withdrawal bleed is induced or not. If it is not, it is evidence that the oestrogen being produced, if any, is inadequate to develop an endometrium than can be shed by the progestogen withdrawal. One then wants to know whether there is gonadotrophin failure (see Fig. 6). This can be tested with clomiphene, oestrogen or LHRH. The vast majority of women with anovulatory infertility, for example, have normal basal concentrations of FSH or LH and it is presumed that in this disorder it is the hypothalamus which is responsible for the failure of production of adequate amounts of gonadotrophin. This may be due to a number of causes, one being a high prolactin level which may be associated with amenorrhoea or oligomenorrhoea. In the absence of evidence of hypothyroidism and any pituitary tumour it can be assumed that hyperprolactinaemia, if present, is an index of altered hypothalamic activity and is due to a relative lack of pro-lactin inhibitory factor. In these women there is a normal basal level

---

1. PROGESTOGEN withdrawal

5 mg medroxyprogesterone acetate for 5 days.
If the patient bleeds within the next 7 days,
the endometrium is oestrogenised.

2. CLOMID (anti-oestrogen)

50 mg daily for 5 days. Wait for 4 weeks for period.

3. LHRH test

Tests whether pituitary is producing FSH or LH and responds to LHRH.

Fig. 6. How to test the axis.

of FSH and LH, but an absence of the pulsatile release of gonadotrophins and an exaggerated response to gonadotrophin-releasing
hormone. Plasma concentrations of oestrogens are lower than one
would expect for the concentrations of FSH and LH in hyperprolac-
tinaemic women, indicating that prolactin may inhibit at the ovarian level although there is evidence (as indicated above) that in the
absence of pulsatile release of LHRH there is an impaired response
to positive feedback effects of oestrogen. Bromocriptine is highly
successful in the treatment of hyperprolactinaemia. Gonadotrophin failure may rarely occur in association with pan-
hypopituitarism, as in Sheehan's syndrome.

A disturbance of hypothalamic gonadotrophin-releasing hormone production is presumed to be the common mechanism by
which weight loss, stress and other psychological disturbances
result in menstrual disorder. Sometimes the negative feedback
mechanism can be set at an abnormal level — either at a too sensitive level or at a quite insensitive level. At a too sensitive level
minimal quantities of oestrogen inhibit secretion of pituitary gonadotrophin, with consequent inadequate development of a follicle.
These patients respond particularly well to anti-oestrogen therapy
such as clomiphine. It may be the case that even when clomiphine
induces follicular development and adequate oestrogen levels there
is also deficiency in the positive feedback mechanism and no pre-
ovulatory surge of LH in response to oestrogen. Ovulation can be
induced in these subjects by the injection of human chorionic
gonadotrophin.

Another defect may be low levels of gonadotrophins in the
anterior pituitary; these can be measured using the gonadotrophin-releasing hormone test (LHRH test).

In polycystic ovary syndrome the ovaries secrete little oestrogen
but relatively large amounts of androgens. This may be due to a
genetic deficiency in the ability to convert androgens to oestrogens.
However, adequate secretion of oestradiol can be induced in these
patients with the anti-oestrogen clomiphine, and this suggests that
the ovarian defect is not primary but again perhaps secondary to
disordered gonadotrophin stimulation. Certainly in patients with
polycystic ovary syndrome LH levels are usually higher than normal in the follicular phase whilst the FSH levels are low. Negative
and positive feedback mechanisms in polycystic ovary syndrome do
not seem to be abnormal in spite of the abnormal LH and FSH
levels. This may be related in some way to the fact that significant
quantities of oestrogens other than oestradiol are produced by
peripheral conversion of androgens in adipose tissue and disor-

dered feedback via oestrone. Clomid seems to work because it increases the secretion of endogenous FSH, resulting in restoration of the plasma oestrogens to their normal ratios.

Thyroid disease disturbs normal cyclical function so that in hyperthyroidism there is an increase in bound oestradiol with a decrease in the clearance of oestrogens and androgens. There is also increased extraglandular conversion of androgens to oestrogens, which again results in inappropriate feedback and a state not dissimilar from that in polycystic ovary syndrome. Here again, treatment of the hyperthyroid state is likely to restore the normal circulating oestrogen levels and normal feedback stimuli. In hypothyroidism clearance of both testosterone and oestradiol is increased because of decreased binding to sex hormone binding globulin (SHBG). Treatment with thyroxine reduces the tendency to galactorrhoea.

The management of hyperprolactinaemia and thyroid disease is relatively easy, as indicated above, but analysis of the endocrine disturbance when the patient's periods are prolonged and/or irregular may be time consuming and costly, and the results of only transient relevance. Practical considerations are likely to be the best indicators as to what treatment should be used in these situations, i.e. while precise definition of the hormonal dysfunction and an attempt to correct it may be theoretically ideal, often this is not possible and the use of clomiphine in situations referred to above may frequently be diagnostic as well as therapeutic. If the patient is not anxious to become pregnant one can superimpose order in the endocrine chaos either with progestogens used alone for some variable period from the 10th or 15th day of each cycle or with oestrogens and progestogens in the same way that they are prescribed for contraceptive purposes. This superimposes an endocrine pattern on top of the disordered pattern and effects what the woman often wants, namely light and regular periods.

It is worth remembering that sometimes the problem is that the bleeding is from an endometrium which has not been subjected to any progesterone influence, and this can easily be remedied by prescribing a progestogen. However, sometimes the bleeding is consequent upon inadequate oestrogen build-up of the endometrium prior to a deficient progesterone stimulus and here it may be better to get back to some sort of normal situation by administering oestrogen exogenously in the first half of the cycle and oestrogen with a progestogen in the second half. It is also sensible to remember that in a young woman stress and emotional upset often play a considerable part in the hypothalamic function: reassurance and patience are better and certainly far less expensive forms of treatment than prolonged endocrine studies followed by complex, changing and often inaccurate attempts to correct the endocrine disturbance.

Further Reading

Gold JJ (ed) (1975) Menstrual dysfunction in gynaecological endocrinology, 2nd edn. Harper and Row, London

A4
Painful Periods

*

Questions

1. a) Have your periods always been painful?

    b) If 'no', how long have you had this pain?
2. Is the pain usually worse before the period, during the period or after the period, or is it present all the time?
3. Is the pain steady or crampy (coming in bouts)?
4. Do you feel it in the tummy/back/thighs?
5. Has it been getting more severe over the past few months/ years?
6. a) Is the pain sufficient to interfere with your everyday activities?

    b) If 'yes', how many days are you incommoded or off work or school each month?
7. If you are having sexual intercourse do you have pain?
8. Before your periods do you have headaches/depression/ feeling of bloatedness/irritability?

9. Have you been helped by:
    a) Pain-killing drugs?
    b) Anti-depressant drugs?
    c) Stretching of neck of womb?
    d) Water tablets (diuretics)?
    e) Taking the contraceptive pill?
10. If married, do you desire to have children at present?

Key to Questions

The questions are largely self-explanatory, defining the severity and duration of the pain and the effect on the normal life of the patient.

Question 2. Distinguishes congestive from spasmodic dysmenorrhoea.

Question 3. Crampy pain is more characteristic of spasmodic dysmenorrhoea and constant dull pain of congestive dysmenorrhoea.

Question 5. Spasmodic dysmenorrhoea often improves spontaneously in the mid-twenties. Obviously, if the problem is improving one should be conservative. If the pain is getting worse this suggests an organic cause of congestive dysmenorrhoea.

Question 7. Pain at intercourse suggests pelvic pathology such as endometriosis or chronic pelvic inflammatory disease.

Question 8. These are symptoms of premenstrual tension syndrome and need to be distinguished from dysmenorrhoea.

Question 9. You need to know what therapy has already been tried and with what effect.

Question 10. Some forms of therapy, e.g. the combined oral contraceptive pill, would not be appropriate if the patient wanted to become pregnant.

The Problem

With regard to patients who complain of painful periods, it is important to get a precise history of when the pain first occurs in

relation to the menstrual loss and whether this is a seriously inconvenient problem for the patient or a minor inconvenience that she
wants to have eliminated if possible. A way to assess this, although
it may not be accurate, is to see to what extent the dysmenorrhoea
alters the patient's normal life pattern. For example, if it keeps her
away from work, or away from school, then the problem is probably of sufficient severity to warrant treatment. If the pain is limited
to the first day of the loss or is maximal on the first day of the loss
in a young woman, generally under the age of 30, then this is the
spasmodic or intrinsic variety of dysmenorrhoea and it is unlikely
to be associated with any pelvic pathology. On the other hand, if
the pain precedes and outlasts the duration of the menstrual loss
then pelvic pathology is much more likely to be the underlying
cause; the treatment of such so-called congestive dysmenorrhoea
must be that of the underlying pathology.

The majority of patients with spasmodic dysmenorrhoea will be
relieved by the combined oestrogen–progestogen pill; in fact over
90% of patients gain some, if not complete, relief. However, it is
wrong to presume that the patient is malingering if she still has
pain of a spasmodic type whilst on the oral contraceptive pill or a
similar preparation. It is important to bear in mind that starting a
patient on a combined hormonal preparation for spasmodic dysmenorrhoea may have its own problems; these include not only all
the side-effects of the pill but also the fairly sure knowledge that if
the treatment is discontinued the patient's painful periods are
likely to recur. It is also important to avoid the pill in patients with
infrequent periods and perhaps also in patients of low body
weight, as both may be more susceptible to post-pill amenorrhoea.
Treatment of spasmodic dysmenorrhoea by cervical dilatation,
which was once a common practice, has gone out of fashion
because of the risk of damaging the cervix to the point that it would
be incompetent in a future pregnancy. Minimal or controlled cervical dilatation is of doubtful value. It is worth bearing in mind when
dealing with a case of spasmodic dysmenorrhoea that the onset of
intercourse and the experience of childbearing are often associated
with complete relief of the symptom. It is also the case that any pain
of whatever origin seems to be less well tolerated during menstruation. Two preparations, one an anti-prostaglandin with the trade
name Ponstan (mefenamic acid) and another with an anti-FSH
function, danazol, have been used with success in the treatment of
each form of dysmenorrhoea, the latter preparation being of value
in congestive dysmenorrhoea associated with endometriosis.

Treatment of chronic pelvic inflammatory disease is initially by

use of antibiotics in women who wish to retain reproductive function, by excision of tubo-ovarian masses if these masses are unilateral, or by pelvic clearance in women who have completed their
families. With regard to endometriosis the cyclical use of the contraceptive oestrogen–progestogen pill will benefit a great number
of patients, and in those not adequately relieved by this form of
treatment the use of a so-called pseudo-pregnancy in which combined oestrogen–progestogen preparations are given continuously
for 9 months (hence the name pseudo-pregnancy) has been shown
to be effective in upwards of 70% of patients. Danazol, an anti-
gonadotrophin, is an effective treatment of pelvic endometriosis,
although expensive and sometimes not well tolerated. New LHRH
analogues taken by inhalation are also effective but expensive. If
medical therapy fails in the younger woman then some form of
limited surgical excision of ectopic endometrium might be considered; if it fails in an older woman it may be necessary to remove
both ovaries, tubes and uterus. Oestrogen replacement therapy is
usually possible without activating any focus on endometriosis
that may remain in the pelvis subsequent to hysteroctomy and
bilateral salpingo-oophorectomy.

Associated with the need to understand dysmenorrhoea is the
need for a proper understanding of the premenstrual tension syndrome (PMT). This usually presents as a feeling of irritability and
almost discontent associated with feelings of bloatedness and
breast discomfort. The syndrome may even present as one very
similar to psychotic depression. It is most commonly confined to
the 7-10 days immediately prior to menstruation and is usually
relieved by the onset of menstruation. It was thought until very
recently to be consequent upon salt and water retention in association with progesterone produced in the secretory phase of the
cycle, but more recent evidence suggests that certainly in some
cases the best management results are not achieved with sedation
and diuretics, a long time practice, but with progestogen therapy
itself. The possibility that in some patients high levels of prolactin
might be responsible for these symptoms is still receiving attention, and there is a small group of patients who are relieved by
reducing the plasma prolactin concentration even if it is not above
normal. It is very likely that PMT is a heterogeneous entity
associated with multiple aetiological factors. Sympathetic concern
for the problem and preparedness to try many different treatments
is advised.

Hence, dysmenorrhoea is a symptom which may or may not
indicate pathology and is of variable severity, inconvenience and

duration, requiring therapy ranging from reassurance only to radical surgery. The taking of an accurate history and careful evaluation of each particular patient are therefore clearly very important.

With respect to clinical findings, congestive dysmenorrhoea may be associated with chronic pelvic sepsis or endometriosis. Both may show fixity and tenderness of pelvic organs on bimanual examination. Spasmodic dysmenorrhoea is not associated with clinical pelvic abnormality.

A5
Vaginal Bleeding After the Menopause

*

Questions

1. How long is it since you stopped having periods?
2. How long is it since the abnormal bleeding was first noticed?
3. Is it heavy or only a stain?
4. Have you had any discharge from the front passage apart from the blood?
5. Do you bleed after intercourse?
6. Are you taking any hormone preparation (injections/ointments/pessaries etc.)?
7. Have you been on any other drugs?
8. Have you been jaundiced recently?
9. Is your urine blood-stained?
10. Do you have any bleeding from the back passage?

Key to Questions

Question 1. The longer interval between the menopause and the bleeding, the more sinister the diagnosis is likely to be.

Question 3. The heavier the bleeding, the more serious the cause is likely to be.

Question 4. Suggests a possible infection in the vagina.

Question 5. This would probably indicate cervical malignancy if positive.

Question 6. Hormone therapy might induce withdrawal bleeds from stimulated endometrium.

Question 7. Anticoagulants can cause genital tract bleeding.

Question 8. Liver disease can cause elevated oestrogen levels stimulating the endometrium.

Question 9. The bleeding may be coming from the urinary tract and not the genital tract.

Question 10. The bleeding may be from haemorrhoids or may be rectal bleeding.

The Problem

The first thing the doctor has to ask himself is whether this woman has got genital cancer, and his questioning must be related to that possibility. If the bleeding has been heavy in a woman some years after the menopause then a serious malignant pathology is very likely. If the bleeding is related to intercourse then the likely reason is carcinoma of the cervix, but if it occurs in a much older woman and is not related to intercourse then the likely cause is endometrial carcinoma.

The degree of bleeding is often helpful in making the diagnosis. If it is no more than minimal staining then it may represent the consequence of the oestrogen withdrawal in the postmenopausal patient leading to senile vaginitis which will usually respond quickly and satisfactorily to oestrogen replacement therapy. It is necessary and important in the questioning, especially in the very elderly patient who is sometimes confused, to be sure that the bleeding is from the vagina and not from the bladder or the rectum. One has to be clear that the patient has taken no form of hormonal therapy; this includes oestrogen creams which if applied to the skin can stimulate the endometrium and may induce a withdrawal bleed. So-called 'flash in the pan' menstruation can occur within 1 year of the last menstrual period and is thought to be due to incidental ripening of a previously dormant primary follicle. The patient is usually quite aware of the loss being entirely like a period and does not present with a picture of intermittent postmenopausal bleeding. Even this 'flash in the pan' type of presentation requires endometrial biopsy and it is probably never justifiable not to perform endometrial biopsy in cases of postmenopausal bleeding. The examination required for all cases of postmenopausal bleeding includes (a) careful inspection of the vulva and of the external urethral meatus as well as of the condition of the vagina to see if there is any evidence of senile vaginitis and then (b) cervical cytology and (c) bimanual examination to determine whether the pelvic organs are normal or not. Any bizarre appearances should raise the suspicion that there may be, as occasionally happens, a psychological factor operating, and most gynaecologists will meet patients who have inflicted injury to their own vaginas and caused bleeding of one type or another. A rectal examination at the same time might be helpful.

A6
Vaginal Bleeding Before Puberty

*

Questions (Usually to Parents)

1. Has the bleeding occurred repeatedly at regular intervals?
2. Have there been any signs of:
   a) Breast development or activity?
   b) Development of hair in the armpits or 'private parts'?
3. Have any medicines, particularly hormone preparations, been taken recently?
4. Has she grown rapidly recently?

5. Has your child been otherwise well recently?
6. Has she complained of headache or eye trouble?
7. Has she any peculiar pigmentation of the skin?
8. Has she had any history of head injury?

Key to Questions

Question 1. Suggests cyclical ovarian activity with menstrual bleeding.

Question 2. The presence of breast development and activity and of pubic hair indicates puberty is taking place. The telarche precedes pubarche, which normally precedes menarche.

Question 3. Exogenous hormones might induce endometrial stimulation and withdrawal bleeds.

Question 4. Abnormal pituitary function may lead to precocious growth and puberty.

Question 5. Rarely a granulosa cell tumour of the ovary may stimulate the endometrium.

Question 6. Probes the possibility of cerebral tumour.

Question 7. Probes the possibility of adrenal pathology.

The Problem

Bleeding before puberty is very uncommon. One initially has to establish whether the bleeding is from the endometrium consequent upon its stimulation, secondary to some ovarian activity, or due to some infection secondary perhaps to the introduction of a foreign body into the vagina. If the bleeding has been cyclical then it is possible that the patient has started her periods, albeit precociously. This is particularly likely if there is evidence of development of secondary sexual characteristics. Children of this prepubertal age are unlikely to have been given any hormones or hormone preparations but if this has been the case then there may have been some exogenous stimulation of the endometrium giving rise to the bleeding. The rare occurrence of a pituitary tumour leading to abnormal production of gonadotrophins is why one should enquire about headaches or visual disturbance. Radiology for bone age and measurement of FSH and LH response to LHRH help define precocious puberty. Paediatric advice may be helpful.

It is obviously best to examine these patients under anaesthesia and avoid distressing them. I have found the use of an infant laryngoscope excellent for inspecting the vagina for foreign bodies in these pre-pubertal children. The mothers usually need more reassurance than their children. Often no obvious cause is found and parents can naturally become disillusioned with one's unsuccessful treatment. 'Medical curettage' with oestrogens followed by oestrogen and progestogen will stop the bleeding if this is necessary.

A7
Vaginal Bleeding During Pregnancy

*

Questions

1. What was the first day of your last menstrual period?
2. Are your periods regular? How many days are there in each cycle, i.e. from the first day of one period to the first day of the next period?
3. Have you had pregnancy confirmed? If so, when?
4. Do your breasts feel sore and full?
5. Are you sick in the mornings?
6. Are you passing your water more frequently?
7. How long have you been bleeding for?
8. Have you passed clots?
9. Have you passed any tissue?
10. Have you had crampy, period-type pain?
11. Do you have any constant pain in your tummy?

12. Have you had any pain in your shoulders?
13. Have you fainted recently?
14. Have you had pain in your back passage when you sit down or your bowels move?

Key to Questions

Questions 1–6. Assess whether the patient is pregnant and the gestation.

Question 3. Recent ultrasound evidence or urinary pregnancy test results would be helpful regarding pregnancy, site of pregnancy and gestation.

Questions 8, 9. Passing clots suggests inevitable abortion and passing tissue reinforces this.

Question 10. Colicky uterine pain suggest inevitable abortion.

Question 11. If pain is a major presenting feature think about the possibility of ectopic pregnancy.

Question 12. If 'yes' is the answer, there is blood irritating the diaphragm and causing referred pain to the shoulders. Ectopic pregnancy has to be excluded.

Question 13. Common in ectopic pregnancy.

Question 14. Again a feature of ectopic pregnancy.

The Problem

Women who are pregnant and bleeding before 28 weeks' gestation are probably undergoing a threatened or inevitable abortion. There are other less common possibilities and in the context of very early pregnancy ectopic pregnancy is a potentially fatal alternative condition. For various reasons ectopic pregnancy is becoming more common in the British Isles and is associated with a rising mortality each year. The diagnosis of ectopic pregnancy should at least be considered in every woman of reproductive age presenting with abdominal pain, regardless of whether she has amenorrhoea, vaginal bleeding or any other symptom. The diagnosis is not easy but if it cannot be confidently excluded, keep the patient under careful observation. Syncope, shoulder tip pain and cervical excitation pain are highly suggestive of tubal pregnancy whilst the absence of any amenorrhoea and a negative pregnancy test are not helpful. A positive pregnancy test with ultrasound appearances of an empty uterus make more invasive investigations mandatory. Culdocentesis and laparoscopy will have to be resorted to more often as diagnostic procedures in the context of a rapidly increasing incidence of this potentially fatal condition. Patients at risk are those with a history of pelvic sepsis or a life-style associated with increased risk of pelvic sepsis, those with a history of IUD usage and those with a previous history of ectopic pregnancy.

As long as you think of the possibility of ectopic pregnancy at least you will not miss the diagnosis as often — though you *will* still miss it. Ultrasound has made its major contribution to gynaecology in the area of differential diagnosis of first trimester pregnancy problems: it takes only a matter of seconds to determine whether the pregnancy is still ongoing or not. In the absence of ultrasound one has to depend upon the history of the extent of blood loss and uterine cramps and clinical evidence relating to uterine size and cervical dilatation to help make the diagnosis. If the loss is minimal and there has been little pain, the uterus is enlarged in accordance with the period of gestation and the cervix is closed, the diagnosis is likely to be a threatened abortion. The opposite extreme with heavy loss, clots, a uterus smaller than it should be for the period of amenorrhoea and products of conception protruding from a dilated cervix obviously means an inevitable, incomplete abortion. Cases between these extremes are best reviewed over a period of time, during which the diagnosis will become more evident, sometimes slowly.

Molar pregnancy may present like an incomplete abortion and again ultrasound makes the diagnosis easy. The urinary pregnancy test is positive in high dilution and sometimes the uterus is larger than is consistent with the gestational age and grape-like vesicles will be seen in the vaginal loss. Sometimes the best clue to molar pregnancy is the general appearance of the patient — 'excessively pregnant' — with pallor and hyperemesis gravidarum.

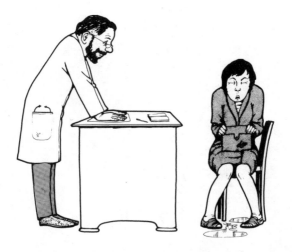

"I can't hold my water, Doctor."

Category B Urinary Problems

B1
Urinary Incontinence

*

Questions

1. How long have you had this trouble?
2. When you want to pass water do you sometimes get wet before reaching the toilet?
3. a) Do you ever wet yourself when coughing, laughing, straining or sneezing?

   If 'yes':

   b) How often do you have to change your underclothes because you are wet?

   c) Are you restricted because you cannot hold your water?

   d) Are you ever wet in bed?

   e) Do you have a chronic cough?
4. Are you going to the toilet more frequently than usual?

   If 'yes':

   Go on to Section B2 below.

Key to Questions

Question 2. If 'yes', the patient has urge incontinence.

Question 3a. If 'yes', the patient has stress incontinence.

Questions 3b, c. Measures severity of the problem.

Question 3d. Wet in bed at night is due to enuresis or a urinary fistula.

Question 3e. Chronic cough exacerbates the problem of stress incontinence and needs to be treated as well.

Question 4. Frequency of micturition is often seen in association with urge incontinence and less often in association with stress incontinence; it is a very common symptom of an 'irritable' bladder of whatever cause (often inflammatory).

The Problem

Urinary Incontinence

The aim of this questionnaire is to determine precisely what is the nature of the incontinence, as stress incontinence is likely to be amenable to surgical treatment, whilst urgency incontinence is not. True incontinence is due to a fistula and obviously requires surgical management. It is also important to bear in mind the possibility of a neurological cause and to exclude this.

Stress Incontinence

Stress incontinence is particularly associated with loss of the sphincteric mechanism at the internal urethral meatus. This may be the consequence of difficult labours or atrophic changes in the menopause, but in more cases is due to both plus a basic deficiency of the tissues. The problem is descent of the bladder base at the region of the internal urethral meatus and surgery is aimed at elevating the bladder base to its normal position. This can be achieved either by a vaginal approach, whereby tissues from lateral to the urethra are apposed under tension below the urethrovesical angle, thus elevating it, or abdominally by stitching para-urethral tissue to the posterior aspects of the pubic symphysis or 'slinging' the urethra up at the urethrovesical angle with a loop of rectus sheath.

Urgency Incontinence

Urgency incontinence is best described as a wish to pass urine which cannot be resisted and is associated with almost complete evacuation of the bladder. This may be associated with bladder pathology or a neurological lesion, although, again, alteration of the normal position of the bladder base may cause some degree of urgency incontinence to be associated with stress incontinence or frequency of micturition. In the majority of these women, however, no organic cause is found for the incontinence and the remarkable feature of management is how rapidly and well the majority respond to an enforced bladder drill whereby patients are only allowed to empty the bladder after increasingly longer intervals of time, starting at half hour intervals and increasing by half hourly increments each day. The majority of these patients manage within a matter of only a few days to hold urine in their bladders for four or five times longer than they claimed to be able to do prior to hospital admission. Unfortunately, many tend to relapse soon after return home. If these patients are introduced to perineal floor exercise so that they learn to develop increased tonus in the levator ani muscles, some continued improvement can be expected. It must be stressed, however, that before these measures are adopted organic pathology of the urinary tract must be excluded by full investigation including cystoscopy and intravenous pyelography. Considerable uncertainty still remains about the normal physiology of micturition, and not surprisingly it follows that the management of some forms of urinary incontinence remains empirical. Specialised cystometric investigation should be employed in many of these cases prior to treatment.

B2
Other Bladder Problems

*

Questions

1. Do you pass urine frequently?
2. If so, how frequently?

3. How often do you get up at night to pass urine?
4. Does it burn or scald when you pass urine, or is it painful in any other way?
5. Do you see blood in your urine?
6. Do you have difficulty starting to pass urine?
7. Do you feel you have not emptied your bladder when you have just finished passing urine?
8. Are you passing more or less urine than previously?

Key to Questions

Questions 1–3. Frequency of micturition suggests bladder pathology, usually inflammatory.

Question 3. Daytime frequency without nocturia suggests psychological problems and removes suspicion of bladder pathology.

Question 4. Again suggests bladder pathology. Pain at the end of micturition is said to be a feature of urethral caruncle; it is not a consistent finding.

Question 5. Causes may be local or general, benign or malignant, metabolic, traumatic or inflammatory etc. Full investigation is necessary.

Question 6. Masses in the pelvis can stretch the urethra and cause difficulty in starting to pass urine, e.g. fibroids, ovarian cysts, pelvic haematocoeles, imperforate hymen etc.

Question 7. Is this due to obstruction to bladder emptying, detrusor malfunction or a neurological lesion, or is it imaginary rather than real?

Question 8. Think of systemic metabolic problems, e.g. diabetes mellitus.

The Problem

Bladder problems other than urinary incontinence are generally the province of general physicians or urological surgeons and are seldom referred directly to gynaecologists. Nevertheless, gynaecologists need to appreciate the significance of these symptoms, though to deal with them all would involve a large textbook of urology. Suffice to say, in this text, that these symptoms would to some measure be understood if the following simple questions were answered:

1. Are there pus cells in the urine?
2. Is there blood in the urine?
3. Is there protein in the urine?
4. Is there sugar in the urine?
5. Are there casts in the urine?
6. Is the patient generally ill?
7. Is there a mass in the pelvis?
8. Is there renal angle tenderness?
9. Are the kidneys palpable?

This is a matter of 5 minutes' examination.

Further Reading

Raz S (ed) (1985) Gynaecological urology in clinics in obstetrics. W.B. Saunders, London

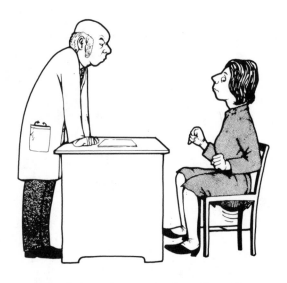

"I can feel something coming down, Doctor!"

Category C Uterovaginal Prolapse

Questions

1. For how long has this been present?
2. Do you have any discomfort associated with the swelling?
3. Does this trouble interfere with your everyday activities?
4. Do you have a discharge from the front passage?
5. Do you have trouble controlling your water?
6. Do you have any trouble in starting to pass urine?
7. Is it worse at the end of the day or if you have been standing a lot?
8. Is it relieved by lying down?
9. Do you have any trouble emptying your bowel?
10. Do you have problems with air passing out of the front passage?

Key to Questions

Questions 1–3. There is often little correlation between the severity of symptoms and the degree of uterovaginal prolapse. Careful definition of symptoms is necessary in deciding whether surgery for a minor degree of prolapse is justifiable or not. Vaginal hysterectomy and repair, with its morbidity and even mortality, is questionable therapy for a minor degree of prolapse in a patient who exaggerates her symptoms.

Question 4. Congestion may be associated with excess discharge, as may decubital ulceration of the cervix.

Question 5. Urinary incontinence may be associated with vaginal prolapse.

Question 6. This is a symptom of the urethral syndrome, and is due to oestrogen deficiency causing atrophic changes in the urethral mucosa. Whether or not bladder emptying is often defective in cases of cystocele is unclear.

Questions 7, 8. Most prolapse feels worse at the end of a long day of standing and is relieved by sitting or lying down.

Question 9. Some patients with rectocele when they bear down at toilet have difficulty defaecating because of the defect in the posterior vaginal, anterior rectal wall, and have to assist the process by placing a finger in the vagina and pushing backwards.

Question 10. This problem is little referred to by textbooks or patients but is not uncommon. It is due to a deficient perineum which allows air to enter the vagina which is then expelled on moving or sitting.

The Problem

Prolapse of the vagina can occur without uterine prolapse, but uterine prolapse is inevitably associated with some vaginal prolapse. Although mainly a problem of the postmenopausal years, it may occur earlier. Vaginal prolapse in relation to the urethra is called urethrocele, in relation to the bladder, cystocele and in relation to the rectum, rectocele. Enterocele is seen in relation to the posterior fornix and contains gut. Vault prolapse refers to prolapse of the vaginal vault after hysterectomy.

The aetiology of prolapse is congenital deficiency of the pelvic floor supports, traumatic damage of these supports, often associated with labour and delivery, and postmenopausal atrophic changes or a combination of more than one of these factors. Symptoms are of dragging lower abdominal pain that is worse at the end of the day, with a feeling of something coming down the front passage. Complete procidentia refers to prolapse of the uterus out through the introitus. Stress incontinence is often but not always associated with uterovaginal prolapse. Getting the patient to bear down or cough will reveal the extent of the prolapse, and the use of Sim's speculum with the patient in the Sim's position is particularly helpful. Treatment is surgical with excision of excess vaginal skin and shortening and apposition of the cardinal and uterosacral ligaments with or without vaginal hysterectomy. Occasionally the patient is of high operative risk and a ring pessary is fitted which provides support to the vagina and uterus by putting the cardinal and uterosacral ligament under tension.

It is worth trying a course of hormone replacement therapy in some postmenopausal women with minimal signs of prolapse: symptoms are not infrequently relieved.

Treatment of vault prolapse conserving good coital function is difficult.

Further Reading

Bloom ML, Van Dongen L (1972) Clinical gynaecology. Integration of structure and function. Heinemann Medical, London, p 262 ff

Category D Abdominal Pain

Questions

1. How long have you had the pain? Is it getting worse or better?
2. Is the pain mainly in the upper region/in the middle/in the lower region/ to the right/to the left?
3. Is it severe enough to interfere with your everyday activities?
4. a) Is it worse at a particular time in your monthly cycle?

   b) If 'yes', is this before the period/during the period/after the period/mid cycle?
5. Is the pain steady/intermittent?
6. Were you ever troubled by a similar pain in the past?
7. Do you have pain on passing a motion/passing water/sitting down?

Key to Questions

Question 2. Location of the pain will obviously give guidance as to the site of the pathology.

Question 3. Pain that is very short lived and infrequent, e.g. once every 3 weeks for minutes, is probably not due to significant pathology — of course it may be, but it is unlikely. So much depends upon your accuracy in assessing the severity of the pain.

So often patients are subjected to negative laparoscopies and laparotomies because patient–doctor communication has failed in this area.

Question 4a. This question attempts to relate the pain to events in the ovarian cycle, e.g. ovulation, premenstrual phase etc.

Question 4b. Congestive dysmenorrhoea precedes menstruation.

Question 6. Twisted ovarian cysts, for example, appear to cause characteristic pain clearly recognisable by the patient.

Question 7. Pain on defaecation may be related to ectopic pregnancy or endometriosis, for example; pain on passing urine suggests inflammatory bladder pathology.

The Problem

Abdominal pain of gynaecological origin is likely to be confined to the lower abdomen. It clearly can arise from all gynaecological organs and be of different aetiology. In practice the following guidelines may be helpful:

If the pain has been present for a long time in a patient who appears healthy and in whom no signs of disease are found on clinical examination, be prepared to accept that no organic pathology may exist. If the pain is of recent onset and getting worse, you have got to find an explanation and there probably is active pathology. This may sound unscientific, but the number of this author's patients who have been cured of their abdominal pain by negative laparoscopy or laparotomy suggests strongly to him that a large element of illness behaviour is included amongst those patients presenting with abdominal pain of a chronic nature.

Obviously pathology is likely if there are positive signs on abdominal or pelvic examination, but abdominal pain in routine gynaecological clinics presents with a frustratingly low incidence of associated signs.

Ultrasound is a rapid, non-invasive, inexpensive addition to diagnostic measures in this area and will prove increasingly helpful. Laparoscopy has enormously helped diagnostically, although some people would argue that it is overused to reassure both patient and doctor and in many cases again reflects the inability of doctors to evaluate pain as a symptom.

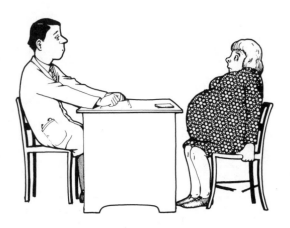

"My tummy is swelling up, Doctor."

Category E Abdominal Distension or Mass

Questions

1. How long has this been present?
2. a) Is the swelling mainly in the lower or the upper part of your tummy?

   b) Is it mainly on the right/on the left/in the middle?
3. Is it increasing in size?
4. Is it painful?
5. Would you describe the pain as stabbing/a dull ache?
6. Have you lost weight recently?
7. Has there been any change in your periods?
8. Could you possibly be pregnant?
9. Have you had any symptoms of pregnancy?

Key to Questions

Question 1. Recent awareness of an abdominal mass suggests that it is growing rapidly and if not a pregnancy may be a neoplasm.

Question 2a. Gynaecological masses rise up out of the pelvis.

Question 2b. Often uterine masses are central and ovarian masses lateral, but this is not always so.

Question 3. Rapid increase in size suggests that it is ovarian and malignant.

Question 4. Pregnancy is not painful but malignant tumours may be, whilst benign tumours are less likely to be painful.

Question 6. Recent weight loss and a mass suggest ovarian malignancy.

Question 7. If 'yes', suggests ovarian pathology.

The Problem

In gynaecological terms a lump in the abdomen, if arising out of the pelvis, is most likely a pregnancy, an ovarian tumour or a fibroid uterus. Having excluded the possibility of pregnancy, the next question is whether or not the mass has the symptoms and signs associated with a malignant tumour or not. Rapid increase in size and pain associated with the mass as well as fixity of the mass are features of a malignancy. The mass in the abdomen may be a full bladder which disappears on catheterisation. A proper history and careful clinical examination will ensure that one makes the correct diagnosis of a gynaecological mass as distinct from some mass relating to the gastro-intestinal tract or kidney for example. However, it can be extremely difficult to distinguish between a fibroid, especially a pedunculated fibroid, and a solid ovarian tumour, and skilled use of ultrasound will make an increasingly large contribution to differential diagnosis in this area.

Management

Because of the possibility of neoplasm, biopsy and appropriate surgery are required unless one is sure that a solid mass rising out of the pelvis is a uterine fibroid or pregnancy.

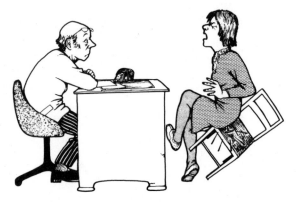

"There is a pain shooting up me, Doctor."

Category F Vaginal Problems

F1
Pain in or around the Vagina

*

Questions

1. How long have you noticed this?
2. Is the pain more on the right side/left side/middle?
3. Would you describe the pain as severe/moderate?
4. Do you have pain at intercourse?
   If 'yes', is this deep inside/at the entrance to the front passage?
5. Are you having difficulty in passing water?
6. Do you have a discharge from the front passage?
7. Have you had any recent injury or operation around the front passage?

Key to Questions

Questions 1, 2. Listen carefully to the answers. Are they vague? Do they change on repeating the question? Is her mood appropriate to the expressed severity of the problem? Psychosexual problems may be associated with this symptom and the more you listen the more you will hear. Ask her to point to where the pain is with one finger. If she can't put her finger on the source of the pain, you may have similar difficulty.

Question 3. Again, are the words used here by the patient 'moderate' or otherwise?

Question 4. Introital dyspareunia is either a manifestation of a psychosexual problem or due to vulval pathology, e.g. tenderness in an episiotomy scar or possibly secondary atrophic vaginitis and oestrogen deficiency.

Question 5. Pain may be referred from bladder or urethral pathology.

Question 6. If 'yes' then pathology is likely in the vulva, vagina or cervix.

The Problem

Vaginal pain and pelvic pain are considered together here. What does not appear in many textbooks is the information that probably many patients who complain of chronic pelvic pain do not have gynaecological pathology. Psychological factors play no small part in this area. If the patient has no fixity or tenderness on pelvic examination and the pelvic organs are normal in size and consistency, she is unlikely to have any pelvic pathology. In situations of chronic pain think of chronic pelvic sepsis and endometriosis and in the context of acute pain, of ectopic pregnancy and some complication of an ovarian cyst.

Pain at intercourse is a separate problem dealt with elsewhere. Pelvic pain may be arising from bladder or bowel or be referred from the back or hip. These possibilities should be excluded by appropriate questioning and investigation which does not need to be more than clinical examination, including a rectal examination and direct examination of the urine. Inguinal and femoral hernias should be excluded.

The older texts made much of pelvic congestion and pain secondary to sexual arousal without orgasm. There may still be some basis for this although withdrawal as a form of contraception is presumably less common than before the introduction of the contraceptive pill and the IUD.

Pelvic adhesions secondary to pelvic sepsis or surgery seem to be associated with pain and division of these adhesions does not always permanently cure the problem.

Post-hysterectomy pelvic pain is particularly difficult to treat and a search for sepsis and adhesions is often fruitless. Sometimes the ovary is adherent to the vault and clearly deep dyspareunia would result.

Pain arises from the ovary in both physiological and pathological states. Many women experience short-lived unilateral pelvic pain at ovulation which is thought to be due to peritoneal irritation associated with minimal bleeding at ovulation. Whether persistence of a distended unruptured follicular or luteal cyst causes pain is not clear, but in the young woman with no obvious pathology and cyclical pelvic pain it is worth suppressing ovulation for one or two cycles as a therapeutic/diagnostic trial.

Vulvovaginitis appears to cause discomfort short of pain, but diabetic vulvitis certainly looks very uncomfortable. Viral diseases of the vulva are sometimes associated with extreme tenderness and infected Bartholin's glands are clearly very painful. Endometriosis is not rare along the line of episiotomy scars and gives rise to cyclical pain due to cyclical bleeding into the scar. Atrophic changes in older women due to oestrogen deficiency possibly associated with some mild infection can cause discomfort in the vagina. Malignant change of vulva or vagina is not particularly characterised by pain.

F2
Vulval Swelling

*

Questions

1. For how long has this been present?
2. Is it on the right/left/middle?
3. Do you have pain or discomfort?
4. Does this trouble interfere with your everyday activities?
5. Does it come on when you have been standing for some time or get worse when you cough?
6. Have you felt feverish?
7. Have you noticed a discharge or bleeding?

Key to Questions

We are thinking here of vulval lumps as distinct from prolapse.

Questions 1–3. How long the lump has been present and the presence or otherwise of pain is relevant. If it is recent, unilateral and tender it is very likely to be an infected Bartholin's gland. If it has been present for years and is not painful it may be a benign tumour such as a lipoma. Inspection, of course, will answer the problem.

Question 5. Excludes hernias but may be confused with uterovaginal prolapse.

Question 6. Infected cysts, e.g. Bartholin's abscess, would cause fever.

Question 7. Vulval malignancy might be associated with a vulval lump with bleeding and discharge.

The Problem

A lump at the front passage is often due to prolapse — see Category C. There are other causes of this symptom and as they may be related to pain in the vulva and vagina they are dealt with here.

Bartholin's abscesses and cysts are common, easily diagnosed causes of this symptom. Marsupialisation of both is simpler and preferable to incision or excision. Masses at the vulva require excision biopsy. Endometriomata are easily diagnosed in episiotomy scars by their association with menstruation.

Urethral mucosal prolapse and urethral caruncles do not usually present as vulval lumps.

F3
Discharge from the Vagina

*

Questions

1.   How long have you had this trouble?
2.   Is it heavy enough for you to need to wear a pad or tampon?
3.   Is it ever blood-stained?

4. Does it make you itch?

5. Has any treatment helped so far?

Key to Questions

Question 1. A discharge that has been present for a long time is unlikely to be a vaginitis although moniliasis may be chronic. Recent development of a blood-stained discharge may be associated with cervical neoplasm or polyp.

Question 2. Some discharge is not abnormal — be sure it is pathological in degree. If a woman needs to wear a pad because of the discharge or changes her pants more than daily, then the discharge is probably pathological.

Question 3. Blood-staining always implies more serious pathology, e.g. carcinoma of the cervix.

Question 4. Most vaginal discharges can cause an itch, but moniliasis more so than trichomoniasis.

Question 5. It is not helpful to repeat previously unsuccessful treatment but the correct diagnosis may be made from knowledge of previous, temporarily successful therapy.

The Problem

Remember how distressing it must be for a woman to go to a doctor complaining of a foul vaginal discharge. Male doctors and medical students might like to reflect on how they would feel having to present with a penile discharge to a female doctor. The woman must feel 'dirty' and often must have anxiety that the problem is venereal. The most likely cause is candidiasis and reassurance along the line of 'this is just like thrush in a baby's mouth except it is in your front passage' is not only welcome but scientifically accurate. If the discharge and vaginal appearances are typical (curdy white plaques in upper vagina and watery white discharge at introitus) then start therapy with an appropriate antifungal vaginal pessary and if this fails follow-up with vaginal pessaries, oral tablets, and lozenges to suck simultaneously to treat the site of the infection as well as other sites from which the vagina is being reinfected. If you are not sure of the diagnosis start on the vaginal antifungal agent whilst waiting for the result of microbiology tests.

Trichomoniasis, if typical, is easily diagnosed clinically because of the pale green blue colour of the discharge and the small air bubbles in the discharge. The classical strawberry vagina is a rarity. Treat trichomoniasis with metronidazole up to 800 mg every 12 h for 5 days and treat all sexual contacts, who should strictly all be traced and examined. *Gardenella* has a pale grey discharge with a fishy odour and is also treated with metronidazole. Not uncommonly women complaining of vaginal discharge on examination have perfectly healthy looking vaginas with no sign of discharge. It is also true that when women with evident, quite heavy discharge are asked if they have any discharge that bothers them, they deny this. Clearly what is normal for one woman is abnormal for another and many who complain of a vaginal discharge do not have any disease but perhaps increased amounts of normal vaginal discharge or some other problem presenting as a complaint of vaginal discharge. It is worth excluding psychosexual problems in this kind of presentation.

Vaginal discharge in the prepubertal child is not always easily treated. Mothers are anxious and this anxiety gets to the child, who is either saddened by it or perversely seems to enjoy it. The psychology of the mother/daughter relationship is sometimes seemingly not quite normal.

Further Reading

Gaya H, Hawkins DF (1981) Pelvic infection. In: Hawkins DF (ed) Gynaecological therapeutics. Bailliere Tindall, London

F4
Itching around the Vulva

*

Questions

1. How long have you had this trouble?
2. Does it cause you to scratch?
3. Does it disturb your sleep?

4. Have you had any discharge from the front passage (vagina)?

5. a) Have you had any trouble with the skin elsewhere on your body?

    b) If 'yes', does the trouble seem similar?

6. Have you been jaundiced (yellow) recently?

7. Have you had excessive thirst recently?

8. Do you pass a lot of urine (water)?

9. Have you had any trouble with your mouth or tongue?

10. Have you ever been suspected of/diagnosed as having diabetes?

11. Is the itching relieved by cream or ointment?

12. Have you had any allergies?

13. Are you on any drugs?

Key to Questions

Question 1. A long history suggests an epithelial dystrophy but fungal infections can become chronic as well whilst shorter histories are more likely due to acute vulvo-vaginitis.

Question 2. This suggests the itch is secondary to vaginitis and vaginal discharge especially of fungal origin.

Question 3. Sometimes intestinal tract infestation can cause perineal itch, e.g. threadworms, and this seems worse at night.

Question 5. The vulval itch may be part of a generalised skin pathology causing pruritis, e.g. psoriasis or seborrhoeic dermatitis, or some systemic disease, e.g. Hodgkin's disease or uraemia.

Question 6. Jaundice is associated with generalised pruritis.

Question 7. This, if positive, would indicate the possibility of diabetes mellitus.

Question 8. As in Question 7.

Question 9. Vitamin deficiency states may be associated with both oral and vulval ulceration and pain and itch, e.g. pernicious anaemia.

Question 12. Soaps and other skin treatments may produce allergic reactions and itching, as may anything else in contact with the vulva, including pants, towels, condoms and ointments.

The Problem

Causes may be general or local, organic or psychological. In practice it is important to exclude a vulval neoplastic change, especially in older women, and to think of the possibility of diabetes in the younger woman. Jaundice and vitamin deficiencies are general causes, vaginitis and chronic epithelial dystrophy local ones. Tights vulvitis has been described and the remedy is obvious.

Investigation includes inspection (which is sometimes fatally delayed in a patient with vulval malignancy), glucose tolerance test, full blood count, vaginal swab, vulval scrapings, fractional test meal and vulval biopsy for suspicious lesions.

F5
Warts around the Vulva

*

Questions

1.   How long have you had this problem?
2.   Have you noted discharge or irritation?

Key to Questions

Question 1. Although vulval warts may disappear spontaneously, if they have been present for months and have become more numerous then you should remove them.

Question 2. Warts may be seen in association with other vulval and vaginal infections, which should be investigated and treated.

The Problem

Condylomata acuminata or viral warts may be single or multiple, spread over the labia, the perineum and even into the vagina. They are best treated by diathermy excision, elevating the wart and amputating it at its base. One should endeavour not to produce excessive scarring.

Condylomata lata, which are described as purplish-grey in colour, are manifestations of syphilis and these patients should be screened for gonorrhoea and syphilis.

Viral warts may disappear without treatment and may recur whatever the method of treatment.

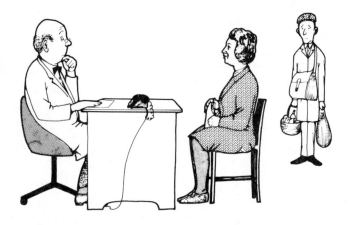

"My husband is very understanding, Doctor."

Category G Difficulty with Intercourse

Questions

1. How long have you had this trouble?
2. Is intercourse painful for you?
3. Is the pain at the entrance to the front passage?
4. Is the pain deep inside?
5. Are you sore after intercourse?
6. Is the pain present on every occasion?
7. a) Are you having intercourse less often because of the pain?
   b) Has intercourse ceased?
8. Apart from this problem is your marriage happy?
9. Have you lost interest in the sexual side of your relationship?

Key to Questions

Question 1. Recent development after earlier normal coitus may be more likely to be organic in origin.

Question 2. Difficulty with intercourse may be due to causes other than pain.

Question 3. Introital dyspareunia. Its causes are quite different from those of deep dyspareunia: vaginitis, vulvitis, psychosexual problems or atrophic vaginitis are more likely causes of introital dyspareunia.

Questions 4, 5. Deep dyspareunia; pelvic pathology more likely.

Question 7. Effect of the pain on the normal sexual activity. It is some measure of the severity of the problem if coitus has ceased in a young couple.

Questions 8, 9. Establish whether there is underlying marital disharmony and, if so, whether it is primary or secondary or unrelated to the presenting problem.

The Problem

The complaint of pain on intercourse may be unrelated to any organic problem and one should consider sexual dysfunction in such patients. It is often helpful for the patient to be asked whether the discomfort is at the time of penetration, deep inside during intercourse, or residual, deep in the pelvis or abdomen after intercourse has been completed. The causes of introital dyspareunia and deep dyspareunia are different. Deep dyspareunia may be due to endometriosis or pelvic inflammatory disease or prolapsed ovaries deep in the pouch of Douglas which are pressed at the time of intercourse.

The causes of introital dyspareunia are more aligned to the causes of vulvitis and vaginitis and one should investigate for such a possibility. There are certain patients who have a so-called dashboard perineum which is consequent upon a failure to incorporate muscle deep to skin in the repair of an episiotomy incision. Some of these patients are clearly benefited by excision of the obstructing skin.

On examination of the patient one should look for discomfort at the time of bimanual examination or tenderness on palpation in the fornices. If, when distracting the patient, she appears to be entirely free of any discomfort on bimanual examination one should again consider the possibility of a psychological factor. One should look for scars that might be causing tenderness and see if there is vulvitis or vaginitis. The usual characteristic features of chronic pelvic sepsis and endometriosis should also be looked for. If the patient has a normal pelvis but is tender on palpation of the ovaries deep in the pouch of Douglas then it is worth inserting a Hodge pessary after anteverting the uterus and then waiting to see whether or not the patient's dyspareunia is relieved. If it is, then this is an indication for ventrosuspension.

Treatment of introital dyspareunia is by excision of tender scars of the perineum and by combating the causative agent if there is a vulvitis or vaginitis. The treatment of deep dyspareunia due to endometriosis or chronic pelvic inflammatory disease is as for those diseases.

Vaginismus is consequent upon adductor spasm which prevents intercourse. It is not, therefore, a variant of dyspareunia.

Further Reading

Craig GA, Milne HB (1900) Sexual dysfunction. In: McDonald RR (ed) Scientific basis of obstetrics and gynaecology, 2nd edn. Churchill Livingstone, Edinburgh

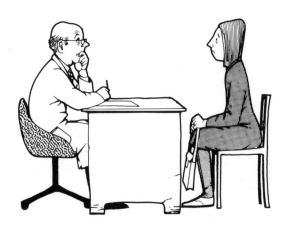

"Why can everybody get pregnant except me?"

Category H Fertility Problems

H1
Difficulty in Becoming Pregnant for the First Time

*

Questions

1. For how long have you been trying to get pregnant?
2. Have you been married or sexually active before?
3. Do you have intercourse:
   a) Two or more times a week?
   b) Less than twice a week?
4. Is intercourse completely normal as far as you can tell?
5. At what stage of the monthly cycle do you think you are most likely to become pregnant: before the period/after the period/ in the middle of the period/between periods/don't know?
6. Have you ever had TB?
7. Have you ever had salpingitis (infection of the tubes)?
8. Have you ever had any venereal disease (STD)?
9. Have you had appendicitis?

10. Have you had any other abdominal operations?

11. Have you had any previous D&Cs (scrapes)?

12. Have you ever had an insufflation test (blowing the tubes)?

Male factor

13. How old is your husband?

14. Has your husband had any children outside your marriage?

15. Has he had an operation on his testicle(s)/hernia operation/ disease of testicles/deep X-ray treatment?

Key to Questions

Questions 1, 2. If the duration of the infertility is for more than 1 year then it is worth starting investigation and treatment.

Questions 3–5. Assess whether there is a coital factor. Even in so-called sophisticated societies coital dysfunction and apareunia remain a significant cause of infertility — not the unnecessary questions that some would think.

Questions 6–12. Assess whether there is a tubal problem. Pelvic sepsis including tuberculosis may cause tubal blockage but appendicitis is not frequently a cause of this. Adhesion may follow peritonitis of any cause and a history of previous curettage may suggest previous abortion and associated pelvic sepsis or intra-uterine adhesions which may reduce fertility.

Thus the questions follow a logical sequence: Is there a problem? How serious is the problem (in terms of its duration)? Where is the problem (coital, ovulatory, tubal, male)?

The Problem

Ten per cent of all couples have an infertility problem. In only about one-third of cases referred because of infertility will an explanation be found. One aims initially to establish that the woman is ovulating, the male is producing normal sperm and the fallopian tubes are patent and coitus normal. In as many as 35% of couples a male factor is responsible for the infertility.

After a full clinical examination and advice as to the time in the month when the woman is most likely to become pregnant, one should arrange for seminal analysis, hysterosalpingogram and a plasma progesterone estimation at days 21–25 of a 28-day cycle; the latter determines ovulation in that cycle. A postcoital test at ovulation should follow to exclude antisperm antibody activity in cervical mucus.

Considerable advances have been made in ovulation induction in anovulatory infertility, but treatment of male infertility is not successful. Management of blocked tubes has advanced with microsurgery and in vitro fertilisation but excessive optimism about prognosis following surgery is unwise if the tubes have been damaged by infection.

Again, patients with infertility require sympathetic management. Although it is wrong to offer hope to these patients where there are no grounds for hope, one should wait until one is certain before telling the patient there is *no* hope. Having said this it is important to realise that adoption as a possibility should not be deferred overlong. Avoid laying the 'blame' for the infertility on one or other of the partners. Indicate that it is a shared problem even if the evidence suggests an obvious cause in one partner.

Further Reading

Hull MGR (ed) Developments in infertility practice. WB Saunders, London (Clinics in obstetrics and gynaecology)

H2
Difficulty in Becoming Pregnant Despite Previous Pregnancy

*

Questions

1. How long have you been trying to get pregnant?
2. Did your last pregnancy terminate in:
    a) Delivery of a baby near term?
    b) Spontaneous abortion?

    c) Induced abortion?

    d) Ectopic pregnancy (pregnancy in tube)?

3.   Was there any fever after the last pregnancy?

4.   Were there any complications?

5.   Are your periods occurring fairly regularly, approximately every month?

6.   Do you have any difficulties with intercourse?

7.   Do you have intercourse:

    a) Two or more times a week?

    b) Less than twice a week?

8.   At what stage of the monthly cycle do you think you are most likely to become pregnant: before the period/after the period/ in the middle of the period/between periods/don't know?

9.   Did you experience difficulty in getting pregnant before?

10.   Have you ever had TB?

11.   Have you ever had salpingitis (infection of the tubes)?

12.   Have you ever had any venereal disease (STD)?

13.   Have you had appendicitis?

14.   Have you had any other abdominal operations?

15.   Have any of these illnesses occurred since the last pregnancy?

16.   Have you had any previous D&Cs (scrapes)?

17.   Have you ever had an insufflation test (blowing the tubes), X-rays of your tubes or examination of your tubes?

18.   How old is your husband?

19.   a) Has he had any operation on his testicle(s)/hernia operation/disease of testicles/deep X-ray treatment?

    b) Have any of these occurred since the last pregnancy?

Key to Questions

Question 1. Assesses the extent of the problem. (A period of more than 2 years since a previous pregnancy despite uncontracepted intercourse, if the patient is not breast feeding, suggests reduced fertility worth investigating.)

Questions 2–4. Relate to any factor in the past obstetric history that might explain the secondary infertility, e.g. infection following induced abortion or a tubal factor associated with previous ectopic pregnancy.

Question 5. Establishes whether the patient is ovulating.

Questions 6–8. Assess potential coital problems.

Question 9. Relates to previous subfertility.

Questions 10–17. Again, assess whether any tubal factor is involved.

Questions 18, 19. Assess any 'new' male factor.

The Problem

Essentially one is enquiring about factors developing in relation to or since the last pregnancy that may have reduced the proven fertility of the couple. Loss of tubal patency associated with pelvic sepsis is the most likely possibility, and laparoscopy or hysterosalpingogram or both may be employed. The questions are largely self-explanatory, dealing with factors that might influence ovulation, tubal function and sperm count and coital factors. Don't be surprised if patients with secondary infertility go for a second opinion if your management is unsuccessful. They feel they have proved themselves so you must be the problem.

H3
Difficulty in Having a Baby Because of Repeated Miscarriages

*

Questions

1. How many miscarriages have you had?
2. What were the details in respect of each miscarriage?
    a) Year?
    b) How far pregnant were you when your miscarriage occurred?

    c) Did the miscarriage start with bleeding, pain or the waters breaking?

3.   Have you had an abortion performed in the past?

4.   Have you ever had a scrape (curettage, D&C) or the neck of the womb stretched (dilatation)?

5.   Have you had a history of unexplained illness or attended a special clinic?

6.   Is there a family history of diabetes?

7.   Have you had much pain with your periods?

8.   Did you have difficulty becoming pregnant?

9.   Have you any history of thyroid disease?

Key to Questions

Question 1. Defining the extent of the problem. It probably is not worth investigating the problem until after the third clinical abortion. Most abortions are due to chromosomal abnormality in the fetus and the spontaneous cure after three abortions may be as high as 60%.

Question 2. Cervical incompetence is characterised by premature membrane rupture followed by a short painless 'miniature' labour prior to the abortion.

Questions 3, 4. Therapeutic abortion may be associated with cervical damage leading to cervical incompetence.

Question 5. A history of venereal disease is relevant and a history of unexplained illness may suggest cytomegalovirus disease or toxoplasmosis.

Question 6. Undiagnosed, untreated diabetes may be associated with pregnancy wastage.

Questions 7, 8. Recurrent mid-trimester abortion may be due to uterine abnormality; this may be symptomless or associated with infertility or dysmenorrhoea.

Question 9. Patients with hypothyroidism do not usually become pregnant, but those who do and those with hyperthyroidism may abort.

The Problem

The majority of abortions before 12 weeks' gestation are associated with chromosomal abnormalities. After 12 weeks mechanical factors, including cervical incompetence and uterine abnormalities, are more common. These may be dealt with using cervical cerclage or surgical procedures. Chronic infections play a small role and are not easily treated. Many abortions may be due to deficient follicular or luteal function in the cycle associated with conception. To date progestogens have not been proved to improve the prognosis in habitual abortion. The uterus seems to learn from experience and pregnancies often terminate later and later until eventually success is achieved. Immunotherapy using the husband's lymphocytes is a recent treatment being studied. The intention here is to induce the production of a protective 'blocking' antibody that prevents maternal lymphocytes attacking fetal tissues. Some success has been reported but final evaluation is awaited.

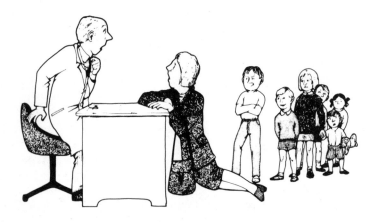

"Doctor, I need help!"

Category I Family Planning Problems

Questions

1. What is the problem?
2. What would you like to do about it?
3. Have you tried to deal with it yourself?
4. Are you clear in your own mind about your wishes?
5. Is your partner in agreement with you about this?
6. Have you thought about the options open to you?
7. Would you like help in understanding the advantages and disadvantages of the options open to you?
8. Are you sure you want any more children?
9. Have you thought of sterilisation or vasectomy?

Key to Questions

Remember the patient isn't ill; your relationship with her is somewhat different. Her choice of method replaces your advised therapy as long as there are no medical contra-indications upon which you might advise her. The choice still remains hers and her husbands. She may nevertheless need help in clarifying the choice before making a decision and the first question she needs the answer to in her own mind is whether she wants any more children.

The Problem

Achieving the optimal method of contraception for a couple at any particular time requires careful assessment. The fact that most of these patients are not ill does not excuse indifferent advice and pre-scribing. After careful assessment a particular method will emerge as having most advantages and fewest disadvantages for a couple in their current lives and relationship. Time will alter the balance of advantage and disadvantage so that not only will the method used need to be monitored but possibly changed, e.g. the pill may be suitable for a newly married couple aged 25 but has little advantage when the woman is a 40-year-old smoker with varicose veins. The variables affecting the choice of contraceptive may be summarised as follows:

How effective is it?

How expensive is it?

Is it safe (side effects)?

How much of a nuisance is it?

Will it interfere with sex?

There are medical reasons for advising couples to have their fam-ily when young if possible. Sterilisation will then close the door on the problem, when the family is complete. Spacing may be achieved by the method of choice but the risk of sepsis with the IUD does not recommend it for this purpose. Anxieties about side-effects of the pill, largely devoid of good scientific basis, continue to grow in the public mind, reducing its acceptability. Careful use of barrier methods at or about the time of ovulation has increasing appeal, as do so-called natural methods in highly motivated couples who have not completed their families.

The perimenopausal years are difficult ones for contraception. Natural methods are made difficult by anovulatory cycles, the pill is contra-indicated by age, the IUD may cause heavy periods and sterilisation may seem unnecessarily radical. Barrier methods may be helpful at this age.

Requests for Termination of Pregnancy

The laws governing termination of pregnancy vary from country to country. The law of the land and personal conscience will influence one's practice. This should not, however, alter the care and concern that any doctor should feel for someone who may be very lonely and frightened. How the doctor responds to that situation may vary and differences should be respected. The patient should not be trapped by a particular attitude so that if she wishes to have the pregnancy terminated unreasonable persuasion should not be inflicted to prevent her achieving her determined goal. Similarly, her fear and loneliness should not be exploited to make her proceed to termination if that is not her real considered and informed wish. Help the patient to come to the best decision for her, admit that the fetus does have rights, if only potential ones, and then help her to do what she has decided to do, as obstructing that course will damage her one way or the other.

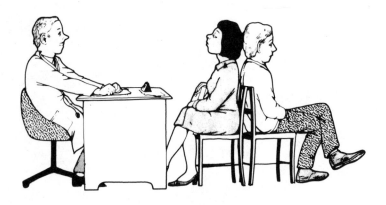

Estrangement.

Category J Psychosexual Problems

Question

1. Would you like to tell me about it?

Key to Question

Question 1. Do not call it a problem: it may not even be a problem.

Don't direct the interview, sit back, shut up and listen — encourage and reassure as needs be, but if you direct the interview, you will possibly go in the wrong direction as far as the nature of the patient's anxiety is concerned.

Leave the area to be considered wide open. Don't close any doors by categorising the reasons why the patient may have come to see you.

Don't pressurise — hence, "would you like to tell me about it", *not* "OK, out with it, what's going on?" She is not on trial!

The Problem

Problems with Sex

There is no other area in gynaecology and probably no other in medicine where a more sensitive approach to history taking and communication is necessary than in the area of psychosexual medicine. Few gynaecological problems are without some psychosexual connotation and psychosexual disorders might result in organic gynaecological disease. This text will not consider those problems associated with psychotic illness.

The important element of communication here as far as the doctor is concerned is to listen with care and sympathy. It has taken a great effort on the part of the patient to have brought the problem to the doctor's attention, and anything less than a very sympathetic hearing of her problems is tantamount to cruelty. The doctor should remember that for many patients normal sexual behaviour is something that they cannot clearly define and it is easy for a patient to imagine or suspect that minor variations of sexual activity are abnormal when in fact they may represent part of the range of most people's sexual activity. In essence very often the patient is asking you to tell her that she is normal. It is as well to appreciate at the outset that if you are not yourself entirely happy about your own sexuality then you should not involve yourself in counselling patients with psychosexual problems. The essence of the best psychosexual counsellors in the author's opinion is plain wholesome common sense. Exotic analysis and complex recommendations are usually of little value. Most women in the western world have had some degree or other of malconditioning with regard to their sexuality and in some parts of the world where there is a more rigid and orthodox Christian practice the malcondition may be extreme. Often, therefore, the function of the psychosexual counsellor is to try to correct as best they can some of this unfortunate false conditioning.

Sexual Activity During Pregnancy

It is clear that most patients remain sexually active through much of pregnancy and sexual activity may even be increased in some patients during normal pregnancy. Most patients do not ask for advice in this area during pregnancy but should it be asked for there are simple guidelines that might be offered based on some sound evidence. It seems logical to advise patients against intercourse during early pregnancy should they have a history of abortion or a threatened abortion in the present pregnancy. Seminal plasma does contain prostaglandins and there is no doubt that certainly in late pregnancy intercourse and orgasm do induce uterine contractions. In patients who have a history of premature labour and delivery it would be wise to counsel against intercourse in the latter weeks of pregnancy, possibly from as early as 32 weeks onwards. There is also evidence that breast stimulation during pregnancy will induce contractions, and again, when there is a history of premature delivery or other pregnancy complications it may be wise to counsel against this.

Sexual Dysfunction

When a patient presents with a sexual problem either as a primary complaint or as a secondary feature of some other presentation the doctor might listen carefully to the verbalised complaint but be cautious about arriving at too early an assessment as it is possible that the sexual dysfunction is multifactorial and many of the operative factors will not emerge from the early discussions of the problem. It is obvious that the husband or boyfriend should be seen, perhaps alone first of all and then with the patient. The interaction between the couple during the course of the interview, which should be largely directed by them, will give considerable insight as to the quality of the relationship, apart from the sexual one, that exists between the partners. It is sensible for the doctor to remind himself constantly that he should not become too directive unless he is certain of the situation and certain that he can do more good than harm by any direct intervention and reorientation of any aspects of the relationship. It is probably also wise for the doctor to help the couple to appreciate that the present dysfunction may be of only a temporary nature, and it is common sense to allow a fair amount of time to pass before feeling that there is pressure to come to some conclusions. A reasonable basis for consideration when counselling such problems is that neither partner has any rights over the other but that they both have responsibilities to each other in their care of each other. If it is clear that love and regard barely exist any longer between the couple, then it is sensible for the doctor not to hope to achieve goals that have their basis in such regard and affection and would not be attainable outside that context.

Non-consummation

Certainly in some of the islands of the British Isles it is still far from uncommon to see patients presenting with infertility who have not consummated their marriage. Patients often do not in fact volunteer that they have not consummated their marriage and this only becomes clear during the course of the clinical examination. The bimanual examination in patients complaining of infertility is often very instructive as to what the coital practice is, and patients who have difficulty in relaxing sufficiently for a vaginal examination who are not virgo intacta should be gently questioned about the possibility that there is some sexual dysfunction. As in all other areas of medicine, sometimes the way the questions are asked is more significant that the actual words used, but it is very important that the patient clearly understands the questions asked, and if necessary one should use direct simple language which the patient cannot misunderstand. When words used are misunderstood or may be misunderstood this leads to embarrassment and hesitancy; the interview tends to become blocked and progress does not take place. Often the best solution in this situation is to change the subject to something at a different level so that one restores an ease in the conversation and discussion and then breaks off the interview. At some later time one can start off at a more superficial level before approaching once again the areas where the original hesitancy and block occurred.

This process of gently approaching a difficult area, feeling one's way, being sensitive to the patient's hesitancy and resistance in certain areas and moving away from or around these areas and approaching them from a different angle is a part of interviewing which probably can only be learned by experience and unfortunately by a series of mistakes and some emotional trauma for the patient. This should not be confused with the difficulty that the doctor himself or herself experiences which is transferred into a supposed problem that the patient has. The worst possible impression that can be left with the patient, however, is that her problem is either of no significance or of no interest to the doctor. It is likely that that patient cannot approach anyone else who she feels is able to help. If the doctor feels that he cannot make progress then he should refer the patient to someone with more expertise in the area who will take on the patient's problem. It does indeed bear emphasis that the doctor must always be conscious of his own limitations, including his own, possibly limited, experience. With respect to non-consummation, one approach that might be adopted is as follows, if infertility is complained of:

The patient should be advised in simple terms that the reason why she has failed to conceive is that she would not appear to have had normal intercourse. One should ask the patient such questions as whether she is entirely happy that she is having full and proper intercourse. The patient in this situation will either frankly say no or she will look a little puzzled and bewildered; at this point one should gently press the point that it would seem from the clinical examination that she has not had full intercourse. This usually results in the patient admitting, perhaps by gesture rather than by words, that this has been her concern and she does realise that this is the case. The next thing to do is to reassure her that in fact anatomically she is normal and that not only is she anatomically normal but you feel confident that she is emotionally normal and sexually normal as well. That reassurance should be a constant feature of the subsequent meetings and therapy. At this stage in the interview I do not find questions concerning the patient's previous sexual experience to be particularly helpful, and it is my experience that a gentle, sympathetic and compassionate but commonsense approach to the matter is the best basis for progress. After the reassurance concerning anatomical normality it is sometimes perhaps wise, as it were, to 'introduce' the patient to her own vulva and vagina and tell her that on examination of the introitus, everything appears to be quite normal.

At the next meeting one should create an atmosphere of quietness and approach the problem again with simple objectivity. By this I mean that the patient should not be treated as anything other than a person with a problem which together you are going to resolve but without haste and without any trauma. It is wise to create the impression that you are going to make progress at a pace that she, the patient, dictates. Any suggestion along the line that you are going to anaesthetise the patient and stretch the introitus and leave it stretched, as was the custom of some gynaecologists until very recently, strikes this author as threatening the patient in the very direction that she feels most vulnerable, and it surprises one that this approach ever had any success at all.

Some patients have been reared to believe that sexual activity is impure and wrong; consequently it is difficult for them to value the genital tract as part of their total selves and incorporate it into their total self-image. The emphasis should be on constantly promoting the idea in the patient's mind that she is anatomically normal and that it is normal that she should want to express her love through sexual activity. It is very important not to try to do more than the patient feels confident to allow at this stage. If this confidence is retained then it is this author's experience that progress can often be very rapid. Sometimes, however, there is a very much more serious problem so that very limited progress is made, and one should be prepared for this.

In practice one method of proceeding is as follows: The patient should be encouraged to introduce her own finger into the introitus and into the vagina and is allowed to get some idea as to the anatomical dimensions, which for patients who have never studied biology or anatomy might be a complete revelation. Some simple explanation concerning the elasticity of the vagina is helpful at this stage. Most of these patients seem to have a feeling that the tissues will necessarily tear and rip open, and the concept of elasticity and ability to stretch seems not to have been considered. Following explanation, however, most patients will accept that the normal structure of the tissues does allow for dilatation without tearing. The patient then uses graduated plastic dilators to reassure herself of the normality and capacity of her vagina. This is done initially in the clinic but later at home with her husband's help.

Psychosis may be associated with sexual dysfunction and a psychiatrist is best able to deal with these cases. Marital breakdown is a problem for marriage guidance counsellors, not doctors.

Thus many psychosexual problems can be helped by listening and commonsense advice. There are few experts, as yet, in this field, and referral to an expert may reinforce a patient's anxiety that there is something badly wrong.

Category K Hirsutism

Questions

1. How long has this troubled you?
2. What measures do you take to control it?
   a) Shaving
   b) Plucking and bleaching creams
   c) Electrolysis
   d) None
3. How often does it require attention?
   a) Daily
   b) Two or three times weekly
   c) Weekly or less frequently
4. Are you on medical treatment with:
   a) Anti-epileptic drugs?
   b) Hormones?
5. Was the development of hair associated with:
   a) Marked increase in weight?
   b) The time your periods started?
   c) Pregnancy?
   d) Menopause (change of life)?
6. Have you noticed any change in the character of your voice?
7. Are you troubled by acne (septic spots on face or back)?
8. Have your periods:
   a) Become less frequent?
   b) Stopped?
9. Are you developing baldness?

Key to Questions

Questions 1–3. Severity of the problem. Recent rapid increase in hair suggests serious pathology. A long history strongly suggests either a constitutional factor or polycystic ovary syndrome.

Question 4. Some of these drugs may cause or exacerbate the problem.

Question 5. This considers the possibility of polycystic ovary disease or changing hormonal status.

Question 6. One of the signs of virilisation; if positive, there is likely to be an androgen-secreting tumour.

Question 7. Acne again indicates excess circulating androgens or increased end-organ sensitivity.

Question 8. If positive this suggests abnormal hormonal status, probably excess circulating androgen.

Question 9. Male type baldness is a feature of virilisation.

The Problem

If the hirsutism has developed slowly over many years in a girl with a dark complexion it is unlikely that serious pathology exists. If the hirsutism is of recent and sudden onset with or without virilism, then abnormal androgens are being produced from the adrenal or ovaries. Define the extent and nature of the excess hair, listen to the voice and look at the breasts and clitoris. Is there an ovarian mass or masses? Check the serum testosterone and adrenal androgen production.

Treatment

Having excluded a neoplastic lesion, do not be too optimistic about the success of endocrine therapy for the as yet undefined underlying endocrine aberration.

Ovarian suppression using the contraceptive pill reduces any abnormal androgen arising from the ovary. Adrenal function and, therefore, any abnormal androgen arising from the adrenal may be suppressed with a synthetic glucocorticoid. A combination of the anti-androgen cyproterone acetate and an oestrogen used cyclically for 6 months has had favourable results recently. The oestrogen is used to prevent ovulation as cyproterone is teratogenic.

Further Reading

Mauvais-Jarvis P, Kuttenn F, Mowszowicz I (1981) Hirsutism. Springer, Berlin, Heidelberg New York (Monographs on endocrinology)

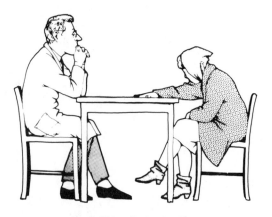

. . . on the shelf, hot flushes, night sweats,
all downhill from now on . . .

Category L Menopausal Problems

Questions

1. Do you have hot flushes?
2. Are they frequent/distressing/getting worse or better?
3. Do you have night sweats?
4. How bad are they? Is your sleep disturbed?
5. What are you periods like? Is there any bleeding between periods or after intercourse?
6. Have you been moody or depressed recently?
7. How are things at home?
8. Tell me about your husband and family?
9. What form of family planning are you using?
10. Are you worried about this or anything else?
11. Have you had any discomfort at intercourse?
12. Are you working at present?
13. Have you a history of womb or breast disease?
14. Have you any history of liver disease, thrombosis or high blood pressure?

Key to Questions

Questions 1–4. Defines the effect and severity of declining oestrogen levels.

Question 5. Intermenstrual bleeding always justifies endometrial biopsy to exclude neoplastic change, and postcoital bleeding suggests cervical malignancy.

Question 6. Depressive illness may or may not occur at the climacteric. The relationship is complex but the depression may be entirely independent of the hormonal change.

Questions 7, 8. See the problem in the broader concept of the marriage, family and home.

Questions 9, 10. A worrying time for effective family planning. The pill is contraindicated at this age, the IUD may cause bleeding and raise suspicion of endometrial lesions, sterilisation is probably overtreatment as the risk of pregnancy is low etc.

Question 11. Oestrogen deficiency causes a dry vagina, resulting in dyspareunia.

Questions 13, 14. Hormone replacement therapy is contra-indicated in these conditions.

The Problem

The climacteric covers the time of oestrogen deficiency with failing ovarian function. This event clearly affects women in different ways and to very different degrees. There can be few episodes in the life of a woman with a greater emotional impact, manifesting as it does the end of her reproductive life and coinciding as it often does with a diminishing role in rearing and responsibility for her children. It seems likely that many women see themselves as less valuable at this time, as well as being less attractive physically and less interested sexually. Apart from being free of the fear of unwanted pregnancy and the nuisances of periods there is little else of advantage for the woman physically or psychologically of passing through the climacteric. Management of the climacteric may improve if these factors are kept in mind.

First find out the nature and severity of the symptoms and allow that they may be influenced by the patient's mood. Then find out the family, social and personality background. Now you will be in a better position to decide how to approach management. Common sense will indicate that the anxious, thin, highly strung woman who says that her life is intolerable will not welcome reassurance alone as adequate therapy whilst a stable happy woman with only moderate symptoms may well be better treated in the long term by not resorting to hormone replacement therapy. The unhappiness caused to a couple by the woman's loss of interest in, if not positive distaste for sexual love, can be hidden but profound. The pain and discomfort at intercourse due to the atrophic changes in the vagina must have been quietly suffered by millions of women over the years. These plus the deeper psychological problems make the climacteric a time when considerable reassurance and support should be sought from all the family. Doctors rightly always emphasise the need for joint consultation with husband and wife in problems relating to sex and fertility and the climacteric is another situation where informing the husband may encourage his understanding and support.

Oestrogens should be followed by a progestogen as the latter reduces the otherwise seven- or eight-fold increased risk of endometrial cancer back to the risk for untreated women of 1 per 1000. No one knows when to stop therapy once it has been started. If the benefits are clearly major and stopping treatment is associated with severe symptoms, then restart treatment for another 6 months. In evolutionary terms, life without oestrogens for women is a very very recent state. Growing old gracefully should not necessarily involve physical degeneration with osteoporosis and skin changes etc.

Further Reading

Goldie L (1981) Psychosomatic aspects of gynaecology; psychosexual problems; the menopause. In: Hawkins DF (ed) Gynaecological therapeutics. Bailliere Tindall, London

Epilogue

At the end of taking your patient's history you should review the situation. Ask certain questions again. It is surprising how often the emphasis changes in a history. Don't hesitate to reassess the history. One would consider it reasonable to reassess a clinical sign such as abdominal tenderness, so why not the history? Beware of inconsistencies and check them out. Get the complaints into an order of priority either in terms of how the patient sees her problems or how you do medically. How serious are her problems? Is medical or surgical therapy necessary? How serious are the risks of therapy? Good doctoring requires skills in addition to knowledge of medical science. Hopefully this text will help to begin the process of developing those skills in a discipline, gynaecology, in which they are essential to efficient and effective practice.

Index

Abortion 39, 40, 78, 88
  habitual 79
  therapeutic 84
Acne 93
  swelling 18, 57
Adhesions, pelvic 62
Adrenal hyperplasia 16, 94
Allergy 67
Amenorrhoea
  primary 15
  post pill 19
  secondary 18
Androgen
  excess 19, 28, 94
  conversion 28
  insensitivity 17
Anorexia 20
Appendicitis 75
Asherman's syndrome 19

Baldness 93
Bartholins gland 63
Bladder
  drill 45
  irritable 44
  full 58
Bleeding
  pregnancy 38
  withdrawal 27, 35
Bloated 30

Bone
  age 38
  loss
Breast
  development 17, 36
  painful 18, 38
  secretions 18
Bromocryptine 20, 28

Candidiasis 65
Cervix dilatation 31, 32, 40, 80
  incompetence 32, 80
  malignancy 35, 65, 98
  pain 40
  polyp 65
  ulceration 51
Coitus
  bleeding 23, 25, 34, 35, 98
  pain 30, 31
Chromosome 16, 80
Clitoral enlargement 17, 95
Clomiphene 27, 28
Contraception 83
  barrier 84
  natural 84
Cryptomenorrhoea 16
Culdocentesis 40
Cyproterone acetate 95
Cystocele 50
Cystometry 45
Cytology 36

Defaecation, pain   54
Detrusor, malfunction   46
Diabetes   46, 63, 67, 80
Diuretics   31
Dysmenorrhoea
  congestive   31, 54
  spasmodic   31
Dyspareunia
  deep   62, 71
  introital   62, 71, 98

Ectopic   *see* Pregnancy
Endometrium biopsy   25, 36, 98
  malignancy   17, 35, 98
Endometriosis   31, 32, 33, 54, 64, 72
Eneuresis   43
Enterocele   50
Epiphysis   17
Episiotomy   63, 72

Fallopian tube
  infection   75
  insufflation   77
  tuberculosis   75
Feminisation   17
Fertilization, in vitro   77
Fibroids   46, 58
Fistula urinary   44

Galactorrhoea   20, 29
Gardenella   66
Gonads
  dysgenesis   16
  malignancy   17
Gonadotrophins   21, 27, 28
Gonorrhoea   69
Growth   36

Haemoglobin   23
Hair
  axillary   16, 36
  electrolysis   93
  increase   19, 20, 93–5
  loss   19
  pubic   16, 36
  shaving   93
Headache   18, 30, 37
Hymen   16, 46

Hyperprolactinaemia   19
Hysterectomy   23, 25, 63
Hysterosalpingogram   77

Immunotherapy, abortion   81
Infertility
  anovulatory   27, 75
  secondary   77
Intercourse   18, 75
Intestines   58, 67
Intermenstrual bleeding   25, 98
IUD   21, 24, 84, 98

Kidney   58

Labour, premature   88
Laparoscopy   40, 54
Laparotomy   54
Libido   18
Ligaments
  cardinal   51
  uterosacral   51
Liver   35
LHRH   27, 28, 33
Luteal
  bleeding   24
  deficiency   27

Marsupialisation   64
Menarche, delayed   15
Menopause
  bleeding   34, 36, 93
  flushes   97
  premature   20
  problems   97–100
  sweats   97
Micturition
  frequent   38, 40, 43, 45
  pain   46
Mosaicism   17

Nausea, pregnancy   38
Nocturia   43

Oestrogen
  binding   29

clearance 29
deficiency 63, 98
replacement 33, 35, 51, 98
withdrawal 35
Orchidectomy 18
Ovary
  autoimmune 16
  cysts 46, 54, 62
  malignancy 58, 94
  polycystic 28, 94
  prolapsed 72
  resistant 16
  suppression 94
Ovulatory, bleeding 25

Pain
  abdominal 38, 53
  intercourse 61
  ovulatory 63
  shoulder 39
  vaginal 61
Pelvic, infection 31, 32, 40, 62, 72
Periods
  frequent 22
  infrequent 22, 27
  heavy 22
  light 22
  long 22
  painful 30
Perineum
  dashboard 72
  exercises 45
Pessary
  ring 51, 65, 73
Pill 18, 25, 31, 32, 84, 94
Pituitary, failure 16
Prolapse 49
Puberty 16, 37
  bleeding 36
  precocious 37
Pregnancy
  ectopic 39, 54, 62, 78
  molar 40
  pseudo 33
Premenstrual tension 31, 33
Procidentia 50
Progesterone 27, 77, 81, 98
Prolactin 27, 33
Prostoglandins 32
Psoriasis 67

Rectal
  bleeding 34, 35
  pain 39
Repair, operations 51

Sex
  none 89
  pregnancy 88
  problems 87
Scrape 19, 80
S.T.D. 75, 80
Sheehan's syndrome 19
Sims
  position 51
  speculum 51
Skin, pigmentation 37
Sleep, loss 97
Smear, buccal 16
Sperm, analysis 76
Stature 16
Sterilisation 24, 25, 83
Stress 28, 29
Syncope 39
Syphilis 69

Telarche 37
Testosterone, plasma 94
Testis 18
Thirst 67
Thrombosis 97
Thyroid 19, 29, 80
Trichmonas 65
Tubal ligation 23

Ultrasound 39, 40, 54
Urine
  bloodstained 34, 35, 46
  incontinence 48
  volume 46, 67
Urethra, caruncle 46, 50
Uterine
  pain 39
  abnormality 81

Vagina
  atrophic 63, 72, 98
  discharge 61, 64

dryness 97
infection 35
itch 64, 66, 72
trauma 36, 37
Vaginismus 73
Vaginoplasty 18
Vasectomy 83
Vault, prolapse 50
Vision, disturbance 18
Vitamin deficiency 67
Voice change 19, 93
Vulva
  biopsy 68
  diabetes 63

dystrophy 67
infection 63, 72
lump 64
malignancy 63
scrapings 68
swelling 63
ulceration 67
warts 68

Weight
  increase 93
  loss 19, 28, 58
  low 32